If Stress Doesn't Kill You, Your Family Might

Words and Wit by Nancy Weil

Grins and Graphics by Sandra Russo

To Dr. R-B,

You bring healing to so many.

Take care of yourself and be well and happy. Nancy

If Stress Doesn't Kill You, Your Family Might
Copyright © 2011 by Nancy Weil

.

ISBN 978-0-9836565-8-6

Published by Toolbox Press. Printed in the USA.
ToolboxPress@roadrunner.com
A portion of the proceeds from this book will go to Herz to Have - A college
scholarship to assist adult women attending Empire State College

It is a tradition to dedicate a book to someone special in the author's life. I would love to do that, but in choosing one person, I fear it will tick off everyone else. So, I will combine my dedication with the acknowledgements and leave those mentioned to sort it out.

Foreword

When Nancy approached me about writing the forward for her book on stress, I quickly realized that I was a perfect candidate for this task. As her boss, I am constantly being put into a state of stress by Nancy's requests (like this one). Her desire to help other people is so strong that she often says "yes" and then figures out how to get it done. This time I am the one who said, "yes" and am now finding myself trying to summarize who Nancy is, what she does and why her message should matter to you.

I met Nancy five years ago in an interview for a position here at the cemetery. The individual we hired needed to be compassionate, organized, a good listener and willing to do whatever it took to get the job done right. Nancy stood out, like always she made that important "first good impression". Over the years we have developed a yin-yang relationship. She opens our eyes and minds to new opportunities, says "Yes" and then tells me to figure out how and most importantly puts the grieving family's needs, wants and desires at the top of the list. She listens and acts from her heart which is filled with passion.

I have been involved in the death care industry for twenty-five plus years. I have worked for companies large and small and have seen the effects of stress in the workplace and how stress can negatively impact relationships, sales and morale on all levels. I have also seen and experienced how stress can affect people personally- in both their health and their overall well being. Attitude is the key element to dealing with stress. When a situation arises in your personal or business life and you let it beat you down, you not only increase the level of stress in your life, you lengthen the duration of time you will put your body and mind under duress.

In sales attitude is everything. Meet someone who has made a living in the sales arena and you will immediately know who has and who has not been successful. The successful person has learned how to cope with the up and downs a career in sales can bring and they adjust with the times. They control their level of stress by always having a positive mental attitude. They do not dwell on the sale they almost made; they are too busy planning the next sale they are going to make.

In this book Nancy talks about being faced with a problem or an inconvenience and discusses the different ways of coping with each. Three years ago I was faced with a problem and, with Nancy's guidance I turned this problem into an inconvenience. After my annual physical and subsequent blood work I was told I had prostate cancer. This is a problem, and with my wife's love and support we quickly found the solution, surgery. Nancy and I talked every day and I realized I could think and stress about this challenge or I could accept the challenge head on, believe in the solution and begin to plan for the many tomorrows ahead, and that is just what I did. This problem became an inconvenience in my life. The surgery, recovery and follow up treatments were just bumps in the road. Thankfully everything went well and I have been cancer free for three years now.

A lot of what Nancy talks about in this book is common sense, however what I have noticed in life is that a lot of us have forgotten what "common sense" is. Nancy drives you back to the basics that center our lives in many ways. She asks you to do a lot of self-evaluation and reflection and fear may be the first thought and feeling you have. "What if my answer is the wrong answer?" you worry. Relax, because there is no wrong answer since there is only one you. Develop a plan. Life is a series of plans, some more involved than others, some requiring more work than others. However if you have a plan, the sudden road blocks that life throws your way are not so difficult to handle.

Now you can read this book or you can really read this book. When a work page pops up, don't turn the page and continue reading. Take the time to invest in yourself. Ask yourself the question posed, think about a response and most importantly be honest. The only person you are going to kid is yourself! Nancy has walked the walk and talked the talk in both her personal and professional life. Listen to what she has to say, internalize the tools that solve problems and decide to be happy by reducing the amount of stress in your life.

I have experienced first-hand Nancy's presentations from both a co-presenter and a spectator standpoint. Even when presenting a topic hundreds of times, each time it seems like the first time. Nancy feeds off the audience and takes them on a wonderful adventure of stories and words. She has now taken her speaking ability and transformed her message into the written word. So sit down in your chair, fasten your seatbelt and enjoy a life-changing read.

As the Vice President of a cemetery I will leave you with one final thought: If you do not heed the advice offered in this book, I will be seeing you soon!

Jeffrey M. Reed
Mount Calvary Cemetery

Prologue

Writing a book about stress reduction, people naturally assume that I live a stress-free life. Right. In fact right now I am typing this in my mansion, listening to the ocean waves outside my window. Hark! I hear a dolphin beckoning me to come out and play in the surf with them. Let me tell you, those dolphins can really get annoying – they never seem to get enough of play time. Yikes! That's it – there is my book in its most diluted form –play like the dolphins. If we could only hang out in the ocean, jumping through the waves, rescuing an errant surfer or two, life would be bliss. Let's face it – none of us live in that world. It is a fantasy – a wonderful, delightful dream.

Since it is unlikely that a stress-free life is an option for any of us, instead, let's look for an effective way to handle stressors before they cause problems. As I sit at my computer getting ready to write a program about how to relieve stress (in my house in the suburbs, nowhere near the ocean), I am applying in my own life the very things I am about to teach.

At this very moment, I am sorting through old legal papers and e-mails in order to respond to an important letter I received. Also, my computer has decided to add to my stress by "disappearing" my Outlook program along with all of my business e-mails and contacts. My limited backup program is not sufficient to restore e-mails that I need to follow up. Oh where, oh where, did my Microsoft go?! Even my 1:00 p.m. client did not show.

Each of these situations has created stress for me, so I am handling it by putting into practice what I am preparing to preach. Instead of my blood pressure spiking and my thoughts scattering everywhere, I am breathing slowly and deeply and developing a plan of action (POA). Soft music is playing in the background, and I am systematically getting organized by focusing on my blessings and working my way back to a psychological and emotional problem-solving place. An hour from now, I will be presenting to a group of adult students about how to laugh more and stress less. It would hardly be effective if I walked in all harried and upset. It just doesn't work that way!

Just because I have learned certain skills in life, I am really no different from you. I do not live a magical life where nothing shows up to challenge me (ask my poor car that now has a dent in it from my backing into a pole yesterday!) Life happens; stress occurs. We decide how we want to handle it!

My techniques do work. Yesterday, three people were questioning my claim to happiness. Each one told me that, "no one is as happy as you say you are. It's not possible." Sure it is if you have to have the tools to access your inner happy, but no one teaches us these tools in school. In all of my years of education, I gained a lot of useless knowledge that I never have needed to use, such as imaginary numbers*. What in the world was that all about? If they are an imaginary number system, why would you teach them? The only imaginary number system in my life is my checkbook balance.

*Definition: An **imaginary number** is a number that gives a negative result when squared. Imaginary numbers have the form bi where b is a non-zero real number and i is the imaginary unit, defined such that i2 = − 1.

Seriously − this is what they tried to teach me in high school math. No one thought that maybe learning more important skills like how to have a healthy relationship with money might be a better idea. Money is numbers – the only difference between $1 and $1,000,000 is a bunch of zeros, right? Mastering those zeros is the challenge. Actually the biggest challenge is to live with less zeros and still be happy and not fretting over bills, banks and investment accounts. Money is not our source of happiness, but it can be a source of stress for many people.

This reminds me of a funny true story about money: On January 1, 1965 Soupy Sales told the kids watching his morning children's show to go into their parent's wallets, find those green pieces of paper with men's pictures on them and mail them to him. In return, he 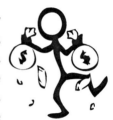 proimised to mail them a postcard from Puerto Rico! In honor of this great entertainer, I will make the same offer to my readers. I am not sure how you will gain access to your parent's wallets as most of you no longer live at home, but if you feel so moved, I am willing to send you my home address.

So back to my theory about school and happiness. (I must warn you, dear reader, that I tend to get very excited about certain concepts and go off on tangents and then eventually find my way back to where I was. For future reference, throughout the book when I detour into one of these rants, I will warn you with the abbreviation R.M. or Random Musing) The only reference to happiness I was ever taught was Thomas Jefferson's writing that we are entitled to the pursuit of happiness. No actual happiness is promised, just the freedom to have it if we choose to. Many people have been pursuing this elusive happiness for years. I know because I hear from many of my clients about how lack of money, lack of time, lack of health and people who have blocked their happiness has gotten in their way. They live their lives in a state of "if only," and they are miserable. It doesn't have to be that way. If we can rid yourself of stress, align ourselves with God, do what is pleasing and avoid what is painful, we can be content and peaceful.

It may take the assistance of a therapist, lawyer, clergy, doctor or other professionals to get there, but that destination can be real. I have been through many difficult moments and I have faced challenging times, but it was on those journeys that I learned the tools in this book, and I am delighted to share them with you.

Once I was asked by someone if I ever have a bad day, and I answered, "no." While I may have a bad hour or two, I don't let situations that are merely inconveniences steal a day away from me. I work at a cemetery and I sit with people everyday who cannot imagine ever being happy again. Their loved ones are no longer with them and their hearts are hurting. Each one of these people teaches me the value of every day and the gift of having those I love in it. Their pain reminds me to savor every moment. They teach me to appreciate what is truly important. Most people are stressing about things that aren't worth losing sleep, health or relationships over. This book is meant to help you understand how to navigate the stress that shows up in your life and tries to disrupt your plans and take away your peace.

Be well and happy,

Nancy

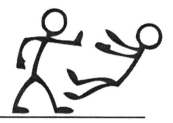

When our relatives are at home, we have to think of all their good points or it would be impossible to endure them.

George Bernard Shaw

Introduction: Perspective

The first thing you need in stress control is an objective perspective, because your ego is telling you that stress is all about you and your experience of not feeling good. It encourages you to look elsewhere for someone to blame. "I wouldn't be so stressed if my boss would just back off," the ego growls. "Life would be great if only my wife would stop nagging me," it complains. "I would have gotten to the party on time if I hadn't caught every red light on the way," it whines. Our egos work us up into believing that we are not responsible for our feelings; life is something that just happens to us. We have been conditioned to expect life to be unfair and difficult and uninviting. We think that life should not be about having fun. Lies, lies, lies!

Life is fun. It can be a party every day. Sometimes the party rocks; other times it may be a bit dull. And, face it, some parties are just disasters. Yet every moment we breathe, we have the choice to show up to the party or stay home and complain. A friend has taught me that there are two types of people in this world: those who take credit and lay blame, and those who give credit and accept blame. It's true; I have never found anyone who does not fit into one of those categories. If you are a blame placer, you will believe that the world is out to get you, even when it isn't. If you are a blame taker, you will believe that life just has to be endured—but it doesn't. Quite simply, to live fully, means accepting that either you choose to react to the day as it unfolds, handling challenges skillfully, or that you don't.

I am a blame taker who is the first to admit when I make a mistake. In the immortal words of Britney Spears, "Oops, I did it again." To err is human, to own up to it is rare. When I admit my mistakes, it leaves everyone around me off guard and surprised, and they have nothing left to say. The finger pointing is done, finished, wrapped up –back to work, nothing to see here, move on. I messed up and I will correct my error, learn from it and get on with my life. No self-flagellation, no beating myself up over it, just a "teachable moment."

So what is stress? We are all taught that "stress is bad." But we don't truly understand why. (Another lapse in our high school education?) Stress is an autonomic reaction to a perceived threat. Once engaged, it can either be shut down quickly or allowed to gain momentum and flourish. Over the long term, unchecked stress leads to the hospital or the cemetery. It also leads to diminished relationships, lost moments and unrealized opportunities. While stress is initially experienced by an individual, its effects are felt also by those around that person. Like a pebble tossed into still water, it upsets the tranquility, and the ripples extend outward more and more.

Stress causes you to change the way you relate to those around you. You may become angry, uneasy, impatient or even rude. Your tolerance level can tumble, and your fuse might shorten considerably. It might not take much for you to start yelling or crying. Pent up emotions that explode without restraint can cause a chain reaction that affects everything and everybody in their wake.

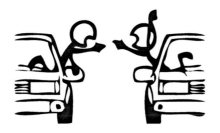

Have you ever been driving when suddenly another car darts in front of you with no warning? You hit the brakes, honk the horn and suddenly feel your heart racing. Your blood pressure zooms up and your face turns red (maybe even purple!). You take short, quick breaths and begin to utter words that are either unkind or X-rated. However, the other car has moved right along on its merry way, and you are actually unscathed, continuing toward your destination. There was no accident, and even though the threat has passed, you are reacting as if it were still going on. Your "fight or flight" center was engaged, but it needs to be promptly disengaged so that you can get back to a calm state.

If you are alone in the car, no one but you is affected by this emotional storm, but imagine that your children are in the car witnessing your tantrum. In one way or another, they are re-acting to your fear and your anger. They hear the string of ver-biage that spews from your mouth (intended for a driver who can't even hear you!), and, if they are young, their reaction may be to release emotion by crying. If the children are older, they may feed into your anger and follow your example, shouting at the other driver, as well. Your stress has spilled over to create stress in those around you.

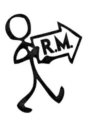

I wonder if they had "trail rage" back in the days when people rode horses. "Hey, your carriage cut me off!" or maybe "Your horse pooped and my buggy wheels went through it. What are your going to do about it, pard-ner?" Or even, "Why do they call it a pony express, when they go so slow?"

The situation described above (above meaning before my R.M. rant) can happen and then pass quickly; the effects are only short term. But what if you existed in unmanaged stress like that every day? How would your reactions impact your family, friends and co-workers? It is not possible to be stressed and happy at the same time. The two do not co-exist. People who are stressed do not laugh easily; they do not respond to change well; they often resent additional tasks that may be expected of them, and usually, they are not good communicators. Stress not only kills the carrier, it also kills the relationships between the person and those around him. That's what makes the ego unstable and unreliable. The ego wants you to think that the world really does revolve around you. "Why is this happening to me?" it whines. The ego is self-centered and it urges you to not

If
By Rudyard Kipling

If you can keep your head
when all about you
Are losing theirs and
blaming it on you,
If you can trust yourself
when all men doubt you,
But make allowance for
their doubting too;

If you can wait and not be
tired by waiting,
Or being lied about, don't
deal in lies,
Or being hated, don't give
way to hating,
And yet don't look too
good, nor talk too wise:

If you can dream—and not
make dreams your master;
If you can think - and not
make thoughts your aim;
If you can meet with
Triumph and Disaster
And treat those two
impostors just the same;

If you can bear to hear the
truth you've spoken
Twisted by knaves to make
a trap for fools,
Or watch the things you
gave your life to broken,
And stoop and build 'em
up with worn out tools:

worry about how your actions may affect those around you. But, like the ripples on the pond, stress affects everyone who is in its way. It begins in the emotional realm but quickly reaches out to affect the physical body, as well.

However, it is within your power to shut it down as it is occurring, which is why it's important to learn how to choose a different reaction. That's what this book is dedicated to teaching. Within these pages, you will learn ten simple tools to knock out stress as soon as it rears its ugly head. As you incorporate these processes into your daily routine, you will find that not only are you feeling better, but you can view life differently. You will be more willing to accept your responsibility in handling interpersonal relationships, and you will begin to realize that life

---

If you can make one heap
of all your winnings
And risk it on one turn of
pitch-and-toss,
And lose, and start again
at your beginnings
And never breathe a word
about your loss;

If you can force your heart
and nerve and sinew
To serve your turn long
after they are gone,
And so hold on when
there is nothing in you
Except the Will which says
to them: 'Hold on!'

If you can talk with crowds
and keep your virtue,
Or walk with kings - nor
lose the common touch,
If neither foes nor loving
friends can hurt you,
If all men count with you,
but none too much;

If you can fill the unforgiv-
ing minute
With sixty seconds' worth
of distance run—
Yours is the Earth and
everything that's in it,
And—which is more—
you'll be a Man, my son!

---

truly is good, no matter what is going on around you.

Living without stress frees you to love more deeply, listen more clearly and laugh more freely. It opens you up to your natural, healthy state of being. Stress is only one option and, after reading this book, one you no longer need to choose. Be well. Be happy. Not just for you, but for your family, friends and colleagues. To paraphrase George M. Cohan, "your mother will thank you, your father will thank you, your sister will thank you" and you will thank you.

Let's get started...

Develop a Plan:

Think about how you handle stress right now.
Jot down a couple of the ways that you currently
react to stressful situations.

Think about what you were taught about life and
what to expect from it:

Think about who around you is affected by your
moods:

Chapter 1

Problem or Inconvenience?

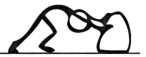

"In times of great stress

or adversity, it's always best

to keep busy, to plow your anger

and your energy into

something positive. **"**

Lee Iacocca

I read a story many years ago in a magazine that has guided me ever since.

An older man was working in the kitchen of a summer camp for children. Working along with him were mostly college students. The food was not very good and the college students complained bitterly as the weeks passed, but not one word of complaint was heard from this man's lips. As the summer drew to a close, the students were curious.

"Do you actually like the food here?," they asked.

"No, not particularly," came his reply.

"Then why don't you ever complain?"

He looked at them and answered slowly and carefully. "You see, I was in a concentration camp many years ago. There, we had nothing to eat. There was no food available, and this was a problem. Here the food is plentiful, I just don't care for the taste of it and that is nothing more than an inconvenience."

Problem or inconvenience? How often in our lives have we labeled something as a problem and justified our worries about the situation because we had to deal with this issue or that event? Yet when we look back on the outcome, it was nothing more than an inconvenience.

Car won't start?
You can get it fixed—Inconvenience.
Car accident with injuries?—Problem.

Computer crashed?
If you backed up your data—Inconvenience.
If not backed up, may be a problem, (but definitely a great learning moment).

Rain ruin your plans?
Change them and make the best of it—Inconvenience.
Flood destroyed your home?—Problem.

Got a cold?
Inconvenience.
Having a heart attack?
Problem.

You get the idea. The first thing to do when confronted with a disagreeable situation is to stop and ask, "Is this a problem or an inconvenience?" When you have that answer, you can make decisions and take actions.

Make a list:

List current situations in your life by placing them in one of these two columns:

Problem...   Inconvenience...

Problems require a lot of thought and information gathering and maybe even a need to "call in the troops," mostly family and friends. When we are overwhelmed and frightened, we need others who can help us make it through.

When dealing with problems:

Assess what you believe needs to be done to resolve the situation.

Determine who can best help, and identify what knowledge is needed.

Do your homework. Collect as much information as possible from as many reliable sources as possible.

Assemble the necessary people, and Ask for help! This one can be hard if you feel that by asking, you are imposing on others, or if you think you can do it all yourself. You aren't, and you can't. Ask for help and accept it with gratitude. Most people are complimented to be invited to help.

Ask God for guidance in connecting with the right people and finding the right information.

Take action. When you are overwhelmed, don't freeze in fear; you're not a deer in the headlights! If you become paralyzed, you won't know what to do or where to start. Mental acuity levels rise and fall in direct propor- tion to the degree of anxiety being experienced. The more upset I feel, the less likely I am to think through responsible, well-considered decisions.

Give thanks. Even at your darkest moment you can still find reasons to be grateful. Focus on gratitude as much and as often as you can. Repeat the following mantra: "There is no storm that lasts forever. Every situation eventually ends. I will survive and make it through. This situation will not last forever."

When dealing with inconveniences:

Inconveniences require a slightly different tactic. You still need to assess and take action, but then you should take a breath and relax. Inconven- iences are not life-changing events, and you will make it through the day. They are annoying, but not alarming.

Last week I returned home from work to a river of water pouring out from a broken pipe in my garage. The driveway had turned to a sheet of ice and the water was backing up into the basement. Immediately I went into action. I found the water shut off valve, grabbed buckets and towels and tried to mitigate the water damage. Once the situation was under control and the water was no longer a threat to the house, I stopped and assessed the damage. The rugs were soaked, but the couch and piano were dry. Some of my books got wet, but the rest were safe. It was going to take a few hours to clean up the mess, so I grabbed my iPod and listened to a book on tape while I worked in the basement. The carpet cleaning company agreed to come the following day to restore the carpets. This was an inconvenience that could haveeasily been a problem if I had not come straight home from work. With a little effort, everything would soon be back to the way it was before, and I was grateful for that.

Full disclosure: Once I shut off the water, the water was still coming in through the vents and pouring onto my bookshelf. I faced a terrible dilemma: Do I leave and get buckets to catch the water and save the carpet and furniture, or do I save my books that are getting soaked? Buckets or books? Buckets or books? I had to make a choice because I was all alone. Tearfully, I apologized to my literary collection of classics, such as:

Six by Suess: I do not like this water break, I do not like it water man. I do not like it in my house. I do not like it by my couch.
Think and Grow Rich: I needed Think and Decide Which – to do first buckets or books?
Life's Little Instruction Book: I went through it, and there were no instructions on how to handle a flood.

Momentarily I froze with indecision. Then I sprang into action by trying to push the bookcase to get it out of the water's flow, but it wouldn't budge. (I should have gone to the gym more.) Realizing the futility of that solution, I ran to the garage and fetched the buckets.

Chapter 2

Identifying Stress

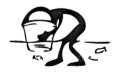

> **"Stress is like an iceberg. We only see one-eighth of it above, but what about what's below? "**

Anonymous

Stress is a lot like love, you may not know how to define it, but you know it when you feel it. Or for my bargain hunting readers, the satisfaction you feel when you get a great deal on those expensive shoes you've been eyeing (you know the ones that will make you feel like cutting off your feet at the ankle because they hurt so much, but they're sooo cute that you have to have them.)   We have all experienced it. Some, only occasionally; others, relentlessly. Whenever I make a presentation to corporate audiences, I hear their pleas to find a way out of the stress cycle. It affects health, attitudes, abilities to function, relationships—there are no areas of our lives that are not adversely impacted when we are stressed.

There are two major types of stress: eustress and distress. Eustress is defined as: stress that is deemed healthful or giving one the feeling of fulfillment. "Eu" is from the Greek prefix meaning good, well, happy or pleasing. Distress on the other hand leads to disease. Again, a dictionary definition: great pain, anxiety, or sorrow; acute physical or mental suffering; affliction; trouble. Nothing we would sign up for if given another option, is it? Yet, frequently, we put ourselves in a position of feeling stressed out, maxed out and on overload. We have all heard about the dangers of stress, but few have talked about the positive aspects of it. To handle stress, we first must identify it.

Eustress	Distress
Motivates	Causes anxiety or concern
Is short-term	Can be short or long-term
Is within our coping abilities	Is outside of our coping abilities
Feels exciting	Feels unpleasant
Improves performance	Can lead to physical and mental problems

Examples of positive personal stressors:	Examples of negative personal stressors:
Exercise	Death of a loved one
Receiving promotion or raise	Divorce
Marriage	Serious illness
Buying a home or moving	Money problems
Having a child	Sleep problems
Taking a vacation	Legal problems
	Generalized anxiety

Judging by the list above, there are great differences between the two types of stress. Physical exercise that puts your body under stress is not a cause for alarm. However, a serious illness taxes your body and can create a real reason for concern.

Planning a vacation? I hate making the plans, getting off of work, doing the laundry, packing, cleaning the house, making sure the pets are taken care of and all the other details necessary to leaving for awhile. Once I am out of town, though, I relax and enjoy every delicious minute of my vacation. As soon as I return, I can feel the stress creep right back in as I sort through the mail, listen to phone call messages, answer E-mails, unpack, start laundry and concern myself with the "details of everyday life." Not to mention having to face the scorn of my cats who were left behind in the care of a wonderful, responsible housesitter. They are sure to snub my welcoming advances and look at me with those cat eyes that say without words, "You left me and didn't even bring me a souvenir." Dogs? They will race to you, tails wagging, so happy that you are home. Cats? They will make you suffer at least a day of penance for your absence.

Let's Practice:

List the stress situations in your life right now by placing them in one of these two columns.

Eustress	Distress

Our pre-historic ancestors were designed to eat or be eaten. They were wired to run from the dinosaurs. There was no time to worry about the situation, only time to react. Today, there is no Tyrannosaurus rex chasing us. However, even when there is nothing threatening us, we still find ourselves in "fight or flight" mode, filled with worries and anxieties. We allow our thoughts to drift into "what if" and "I should have," and it is our thoughts that allow stress to remain in control.

Have you ever wakened from a sound sleep, worried and fearful about something that never actually happened? I have. I used to be a terrific worrier. I could lose sleep over what the weather was going to do the next day—as if I had any control over the weather. If it snowed, then the patients would cancel, and we would not be able to make a deposit. That would mean not being able to make payroll. However, the reality was that even if it did snow, we always made payroll, and the bills always got paid.

My fear about lack of money used to be enormous. I stressed more about that than anything else. One day, as I was ruminating over my lack of funds, the proverbial "light bulb" went on over my head. What if I took this to its most absurd conclusion? I began to ask myself a list of questions:

Had I ever not had food to eat?
No.
Had the utilities ever been shut off for lack of payment?
No.
Had I ever not been able to put gas in my car?
No.
Did my children have clothes to wear?
Yes.

The list went on and on, presenting every possible outcome that lack of money could bring. Finally I realized that though I may not have had extra money in the bank, I always had enough to cover the essentials, so I began to relax. My shadowy fears were unfounded. The things I worried about the most never occurred, and it was unlikely they would start to occur now. Content with my answer, I was able to fall back to sleep—in my own house, with clean sheets on the bed, wearing comfy pajamas…you get the picture. I really did not lack for anything.

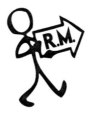

Since anxiety around money is common for so many people, I want to share with you an epiphany I had. Some people are constantly afraid that they do not have enough money to pay for their needs. There is never enough money is a common thought pattern. And it is true, for what you focus on, you get more of. Pay attention to that gem of my philosophy of life that I just shared with you: What you focus on, you get more of. So, if you believe that you never have enough money, you will continue to not have enough money.

Some people pride themselves on always having "just enough." If an unexpected bill comes up, these folks will somehow find a way to pay it. The money shows up in the amount they need to cover every anticipated and unanticipated expense. It is like a mini-miracle for them. Car breaks down? Someone who has owed you money for years suddenly decides to mail you a check and it is for the same amount as the repair shop's estimate. While "just enough" won't fill your bank account, your 401K or your rainy day fund, you'll get by, but you will always continue to wonder how you'll make it through the month.

Finally, there are people just attract money. They expect to have it, they are not afraid to work for it (and to charge for what they are worth) and they are not ashamed to have money. They love the life that money provides for them. Many are generous and charitable and spread the wealth to worthy causes. Right now you are probably picturing Bill Gates or Arnold Palmer, but I know people who thrive, even on minimum wage jobs. They still put money away for a rainy day, travel, donate to charities and live life fully and happily.

Money is just a number with a bunch of zeros attached (remember?) and the amount to make us happy changes with your circumstances and attitude. In some parts of the world, the average yearly income is less than $1,000. If a person from one of these countries moves to the United States and gets a minimum wage job, their income rises more than fourteen times. They would consider themselves very wealthy, wouldn't they? But it's all about perspective and attitude. Money is only what we exchange with one another to provide for our needs and wants. If you want to erase your money worries, then first

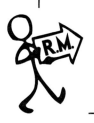

understand how you view money. While it can be an important thing to have, it is not worth losing your life over (but some people do following every Wall Street crash.)

Chapter 3

Stress Triggers

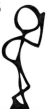

"If you asked,
'what is the single most important
key to longevity?'
I would have to say it is avoiding
worry, stress and tension.
And if you didn't ask me, I'd still
have to say it. "

George Burns

It seems to me that the easiest way to avoid stress is to figure out what causes it and then avoid those things. We all have people, situations or events that trigger stress reactions in us. Some people have them so much of the time that they no longer know what calm feels like!

I have met people who are addicted to drama. They feed off the warped excitement of the situation and love to tell the story to anyone who will listen. It doesn't matter if they are retelling their own lives or someone else's tragedy, they just love to gossip about the high drama in the situation. Sometimes these folks act like the victim in the story, "Why does this always happen to me?," they cry. Other times, they assume the role of rescuer, "I don't know what they would have done if I had not been there." They are always getting a payoff (gain) for their efforts.

For people who are addicted to drama, even negative consequences are acceptable. It's a vicious cycle, and "feeling good" can never be achieved. If this describes you on any level, ask yourself what you are you getting from this. I have asked many clients this question, and their answers have amazed me. Sometimes they look incredulous and assume I did not hear their story clearly. Certainly they were the victims with no personal benefit at all in the melodrama. Sometimes, though, they will look deeper and see how they gain in replaying the role again and again.

Drama addicts are not about a single episode or event where bad things happen. The type of drama I am describing is when the behavior becomes a negative pattern in a person's life. In order for the person to move forward and find peace, the cycle must be broken. Sometimes it is just a matter of being aware of the pattern and then stopping it as soon as it starts. Other times, professional help is needed to overcome a lifetime of habit. The bottom line is that it is not possible to find serenity while seeking the continual adrenaline rush of drama.

Stress triggers are predictable. Mary relates that every time she looks at the pile of unopened mail sitting on her table, she feels overwhelmed. Stress accompanies John to his office each day as he gets to his desk and sees the unfinished projects. Howard, on the other hand, hates when his well-planned day suddenly takes an unexpected turn: a cancelled appointment, a client who shows up late, a last-minute addition to his "to do" list. Everyone has something or someone that triggers stress.

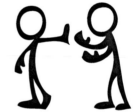

Now, replace "mother-in-law" with the name of the person who most gets your goat. Is it a relative, a co-worker, a friend (or former friend)? Is there someone in your life who gets you upset even if you just think about them, not to mention being around them? If it is possible to avoid those people altogether, problem solved. But if it's your boss, for instance, you must interact, and the stress begins before you even see him/her.

> **M**y mother-in-law is a well-balanced person. She's got a chip on both shoulders.

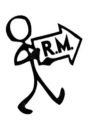

I looked up the origin of the expression, **"gets your goat." While there is some argument that this is merely an urban legend, I think there is a good lesson within the tale. It is claimed that the expression comes from an old horse-racing practice. A goat was said to have a**

This is an excellent example of giving away your power. When you allow someone else to control your peace of mind or your ability to function at your best, you have given them your power. Eleanor Roosevelt said, "No one can make you feel inferior without your consent," but I would add, "No one can make you feel stressed without your consent."

You can feel however you want to feel; that is part of your power. No one but you is in control of your emotions. There is not a person on this planet who has the power to make you upset, if you choose not to buy into their behavior. The Dalai Lama tells the story of a formerly imprisoned Buddhist monk who became afraid for his life during his incarceration. When asked why he was afraid, he replied that he was starting to lose compassion for his jailers. Imagine being wrongly imprisoned, yet maintaining compassion for those who keep you locked up. Nelson Mandela did. So did Mahatma Gandhi. What was it within them that allowed them to not become bitter towards others? Can we access that gift, too?

Many years ago (before I was so highly evolved), my best friend taught me this lesson in a powerful way. I was a volunteer for an organization and the person who ran the office was what I now call a "crazy maker." Just a comment from her could push my buttons and upset me. One day, when she had been partic-

---

calming effect on the high-strung horses. Prior to the race, a goat was kept in the stall with the thoroughbred. If someone wanted to throw the race, they would steal the goat. That would upset the horse, causing it to run a bad race. So if someone has "gotten your goat" they are somehow upsetting you and disrupting your ability to think and act clearly.

ularly adept at "getting my goat," I left her office, enraged. My head was pounding; my blood pressure was through the roof; I was steaming mad. Later, when I called my friend and told her all that this woman had done to upset me, she listened calmly and then asked a very simple question, "Does she have anyone who loves her?"

After I thought about it for a moment, I replied, "She must. She has a husband, children and grandchildren. What is your point?"

Her answer has guided me ever since. "Then she must be lovable; you have just not found that part in her yet." So, if you have "crazy makers" in your life who stress you out, steal your bliss and upset you, try to find that part in them that is lovable. Great Hollywood movies are written around this very theme—*The Devil Wears Prada* and *The Proposal*, for instance. We are multi-dimensional beings who should not judge or be judged too quickly.

By the way, in case you are wondering whatever happened to the crazy maker I referenced above, I never did find that lovable place in her. She was fired and I was happy. The End.

> **66 She was fired and I was happy. 99**

It is not easy to overcome negativity with calm. We may not be capable at all times of being like the Dalai Lama or Mother Teresa. We can, however, work toward that goal and practice not buying in to other's attitudes and actions. We can be more serene and less stressed no matter whom we are around.

Stress triggers must be recognized. Willy Wonka put it best when he said, "So much time, and so little to do. Wait a minute. Strike that; reverse it." Before you can prevent stress from getting started, you must recognize what creates stress for you. Then avoid those situations by putting into place actionable steps that allow you to remain in control and stress free.

Write down your stress triggers:

Chapter 4

Know Thyself

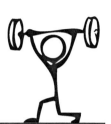

66 If your teeth are clenched

and your fists are clenched,

your lifespan

is probably clenched. 99

Terri Guillemets

Stress that remains unchecked over time leads to disease. Your body will give you fair warning when it is stressed, so you can listen to its message and redirect your response. You could also just ignore the warnings and end up forced to rest due to illness or disease or even death. Stress related conditions include:

- Heart disease
- Stroke
- Digestive problems
- Headaches
- Sexual dysfunction
- High blood pressure…and the list goes on and on.

It is imperative to get up-close-and-personal with your physical body. (Get your mind out of the gutter and stop your middle school giggling right now.) It has an intelligence of its own (Hmmm, maybe my physical body understands the imaginary number system) and a very sophisticated emergency warning system (Mine screams, "Danger Will Robinson"). How often do you get quiet enough to "check in" with your body? When you become aware that it's out of sorts, do you ignore it and keep pushing ahead with your agenda, or do you feed it well, rest it enough and exercise it regularly? How do you honor this structure that carries you around all day and does your bidding for you? I have found that a trip to Dessert Deli does wonders for my attitude and allows me to take a much needed break. Until something goes wrong, we rarely notice our bodies. Then it is all we notice! Wouldn't it be better to pay attention before it's too late?

Lloyd enjoyed his job. Although he worked long hours and the pay was never great, he felt deep satisfaction in keeping his company profitable. He liked his clients and most of his co-workers. He liked his job so much that he was rarely at home with his wife and kids. He was determined that providing for his family was the best way he could show them his love and prove that he cared about them. Why else would I work this hard? he wondered. But then the cancer came along, and everything changed. Cancer treatments made him too weak to work. He had to stay home and rely on the very people he had ignored for so long. Faithful friends stopped by to keep his spirits up, and his devoted family accompanied him to every doctor's appointment and chemo treatment. Cancer had become a new member of his family.

But instead of appreciation, the situation made Lloyd extremely angry. Cancer was robbing him of the life he had known and loved. Each day he grew a little bit weaker and a little bit sicker. Facing his own mortality, Lloyd suddenly had an epiphany. He realized that there were only two possible outcomes to this diagnosis. Either he would die, and his problems would end, or he would live and never be the same again. No longer could work take center stage. When he realized how important friends and family had become to him, the idea of spending long hours at the office no longer appealed to him. If he survived, he knew what mattered most and he would not go back to living the way he had before. Cancer had changed him and he was grateful for the lesson that taught him what was truly important to him. Lloyd began to bless the cancer! With his newfound awareness, he completely healed and lived a happier life.

It isn't necessary to get cancer in order to become aware of what is important in your life. You also don't have to get cancer in order to become aware of how important your health is to your well being. When you are stressed, your body tells you about it pretty quickly. You might get a tension headache or your stomach may turn flip flops. You either can't eat or you eat every sugary, carb-loaded tidbit in sight. Do you feel as if there's a pit in your stomach? Is your heartbeat racing? Are you taking shallow breaths or feeling your muscles tightening? How often do you wake up in the middle of the night with your anxieties on high alert? Are your shoulders touching your earlobes? Stress is a physical clue to the manifestation of emotional issues. Pay attention—before it's too late.

Make another list:

List all of the ways that stress shows up in your body (i.e. headache, muscle tension, upset stomach, etc.)

In Other Words...

Let's sum up everything we've studied so far:
The three simple steps to stress relief are: State it, Rate it, Obliterate it.

State it: Notice the signs when you are getting stressed. Awareness is necessary in order to handle stress. We live in a stressed condition so much of the time, sometimes we are not even aware of it until it becomes unmanageable or we get sick. There are two ways to notice stress early. The first is just a simple statement of observation: I am stressed at this moment. The second is to delve a little deeper and determine what is triggering the stress. I am stressed right now because I have a deadline for this project. I am not yet finished, and I'm worried that I won't get it done on time. I suppose there is a third way as well. This is when you are plucking your eyebrows out one by one and mumbling to yourself about needing to visit the wizard.

Rate it: How powerful is the stress? Is it merely an annoyance, or is your blood pressure off the chart? Different levels of stress require different approaches. Low stress levels may just need a moment of calm breathing, but unrelenting stress may send you to the doctor or therapist. Extreme stress can also

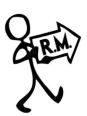

I believe that if you are going to take a day off of work, it should not be because you are sick or stressing out. I think everyone should be allowed to take at least one day off each year as an "I am feeling too good to come to work today" day. You know those days when the sun is shining and you are feeling great and you fear that showing up at the office might just bring cause you to over-react in certain situations. The dog throws up on your new carpet, the car won't start and forcing you to be late for work. What you might be able to handle on "good" days can send you over the edge if the stressors are allowed to build up. Suddenly you are yelling at the dog, cursing the car and taking the entire day off of work rather than showing up a little late. By rating your stress, you are able to get a handle on it before it overtakes you and leaves you unbalanced.

Obliterate it: Dispatch that stress as quickly as possible. Understand these tools, practice with them until they are part of your "automatic reaction," and have a plan of action you have practiced in advance. Then, stress won't get to rule your day and steal your peace. Do you want to thrive or just survive? You don't have to become a ninja warrior of stress relief, just a few simple tools and none of them involve Ninja throwing stars. Hmmm, that gives me a branding idea, Nancy Weil – Ninja Warrior of Stress Relief.

You have already learned steps one and two, so let's move on to step three. How to obliterate stress...

you down. *HR managers:* remember my philosophy of life: You get more of what you focus on. So if you only offer sick days, then you will have sick employees. *Employees:* Get real. You know that you are doing this anyway, so wouldn't it be great if you didn't have to fake a cough and a sad, little sick voice and could just call up your boss and say, "I'm calling in well today. I feel amazing and don't want to have work bring me down, so I'll see you tomorrow."

Chapter 5

Ten Tools for Stress Relief

" There are very few certainties that touch us all in this mortal experience, but one of the absolutes is that we will experience hardship and stress at some point. "

Dr. James C. Dobson

In this section you will discover ten tools you can use to get rid of stress immediately. You don't have to wait for the situation to change or any other external stimuli to pass. You have the power to conquer stress in the moment by having a plan. Once you have mastered the tools, you are not powerless over stress. By using these techniques you can relax and get back to a calm state.

At the end of each of my laughter clubs, after we have been laughing together for forty-five minutes, I ask everyone to sit down, close their eyes and become aware of how they are feeling. Most report that their legs are tingling, their breathing is deeper and they feel more alert. They are completely relaxed, yet totally energized.

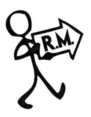

I have the distinction of running the only laughter club held at a cemetery anywhere in the world. At any given gathering, I am joined by the bereaved, people who are looking to laugh more, a couple of clowns and a group of nuns. You have not fully lived until you have spent an evening laughing with nuns. They are such wonderful souls and add so much to our group. I mention this because nuns are often unfairly maligned as stern looking old ladies armed with rulers. My nuns wear clown noses and are armed with imaginary lawn mowers.

Imagine that feeling. You are alert and your brain is awake, yet there is no tension in your muscles, your thoughts or your body. This is your natural state of being, it is the way your body was designed originally. We were not intended to be in a continual state of stress, fight or flight. We are not designed to be tired, apathetic or depressed. We are energy beings and our energy is supposed to feel good. We just have to let go of what weighs us down and uncover what is already present.

In order to harness the power of these tools, you should first read through them all. Then focus on the ones that most resonate with you. Which ones are you most likely to use? Under what circumstances would you use them? Do you have the materials needed in order to implement your plan? Are you armed with your Ninja journals or Ninja pedometer? Nancy Weil-Ninja Warrior of Stress Relief has these products and more available through my website (not really.)

Like any new behavioral change, you must first start with a determination to change your reactions to stress. Then you need to write down your Stress Plan of Action (SPOA). Be sure you have on hand the items you need in order to use the stress-reduction tools. Then be alert to the need to utilize the plan.

At first, you may slip and allow yourself to fall back into old patterns. Don't berate yourself, just notice and decide to act differently the next time the trigger occurs. It is important that you have a plan in place before stress occurs. That way you are not caught unprepared.

One evening on my way to give a program on the healing benefits of laughter to an organization that helps sick children, I knew the volunteers in the audience needed an emotional boost. They were run down, and compassion fatigue was setting in. The organization had lost some valuable volunteers who just could not continue to work with the children and their families. I needed to be "up" and ready to re-energize them and help them approach their jobs with a renewed commitment to the families they served as well as to their own self care.

With time to spare before I arrived, the unexpected happened. I got caught in a hopeless traffic jam due to an accident. Nothing was moving! Sitting in my car about a mile away from the next exit, it might as well have been a hundred miles away, because clearly I wasn't going anywhere!

Naturally, I could feel my stress level rise as I thought about the people who would be wondering where the speaker was. I also realized that showing up late, stressed and frustrated, would not be conducive to a program on laughter and healing. Nor could I be any kind of role model for my own teaching. So I put into action my rehearsed plan for just such a situation. I called the organizer and explained my predicament so that she knew I would be there as soon as I could.

Next I reached into my glove compartment and put on my clown nose. I have found it impossible to feel stressed while wearing a clown nose—you just feel stupid being angry when wearing one! Next, I grabbed a stress ball and began to squeeze it. I tuned my radio to a soothing classical station, and I chose to relax. A few deep breaths later reminded me that if I was stuck in this traffic jam so are some of the people on the way to the talk. Gradually, I made my way to the next exit, wound through back streets and arrived at my destination, late but ready to roll. The program turned out great and I was well received—especially because I walked in still wearing my red nose.

Let's think about a
Stress Plan of Action (SPOA)

How do you currently react to stress? What do you do to reduce it? Maybe you already have the beginning of an SPOA?

I react to stress by:

To reduce stress, I:

Chapter 6

Tool 1: Take a Breath

" Stress is basically a disconnection from the earth, a forgetting of the breath. **"**

Natalie Goldberg

Remember when you were a child and you got all excited about something? This happened to me whenever I heard the magical music that announced that Mr. Charley was coming. We didn't have Mr. Softee® in my neighborhood, instead we had a drunken old man who disliked children, but drove around with a truck filled with ice cream and candy. We loved Mr. Charley. Back to your memories of childhood, when you went running up to your mother and she would put out her hand and say, "Slow down a minute and take a breath"? Breathing—the basis of all life. When we are born, we draw our first breath and when we die, we draw our last. In between, we take millions of breaths. To calculate how many you have taken so far, check out this cool website:

www.health.discovery.com/centers/heart/beatsbreaths/beats breaths.html

Since the number of breaths per hour varies depending on age, activity and health factors, let's just say we average nine hundred breaths per hour or fifteen breaths per minute. Most of the time, we don't even notice our breathing, unless we are out of breath or having trouble inhaling. Notice the words we use to describe our breathing:

When we exercise, we get *out* of breath.
If we need a break, we *catch* our breath.
A beautiful sight or feeling *takes away* our breath.

All of these phrases use action words, yet none of them are calming or refer to the abundance of breaths we take. We fear losing our breath, even though we breathe over twenty-thousand times a day! For something so necessary to our well-being, we don't pay enough attention to it. I work at a cemetery, and believe me when I say that I think breathing is very important! When you stop breathing, I may meet you at my place of business.

If you're thinking, I breathe all day long, so what is the big deal? How can this help me get through the day? Even though we breathe all day, we don't do it mindfully. We need to begin to breathe again the way infants naturally breathe—from the diaphragm. Other than an occasional wet diaper or hunger, babies have no stress, so they breathe from deep within their lungs. With each breath, their bellies rise and fall slowly. Adults, on the other hand, stress breathe. Shoulders hunch up and down with each breath and only the top of our lungs fill with fresh oxygen.

Let's try a breathing exercise:

Place one hand on your chest and one on your belly. Take a few breaths and notice which hand is moving.

If it is your upper hand, you are stress breathing.

The lower hand indicates that you are breathing deeply from the diaphragm.

The middle hand indicates that you are standing way too close to someone and they should get their hand off of you right now or they'll distract you from this important exercise!

The hand that moved is:

At times of stress, we usually take short, quick breaths. In order to regain our calm center, we need to focus on our breathing. It's really quite simple once you know how. There are many breathing techniques, but I will introduce you to only four of them (A yoga instructor tried to teach me the Breath of Fire, but I am afraid of flames, so it didn't work out). Some can be done silently with no one around aware of what you are doing. Others you may want to do when you are alone. Each is effective at giving you the result you want—less stress in the moment.

Technique #1 – The 4-4-4 Breath

Back-to-basics breathing is simple and effective. It can be done anywhere, anytime, in any way.
Inhale while counting to four very slowly.
Hold your breath for a slow count of four.
Exhale to a very slow count of four.
Five to ten cycles of this exercise should leave you feeling calm and refreshed.

Technique #2 – Alternate Nostril Breathing

This is a technique taught to me by a yoga instructor. It is very effective, but you may not want to do this in front of other people!
With your thumb, close the right nostril and inhale deeply.
Still keeping nostril closed, exhale completely.
Using your ring finger, close the left nostril. Leave the right nostril open and inhale deeply.
With left nostril still closed, exhale completely.
Repeat cycle three or four times until you feel calm and relaxed.

Note: An alternative to this is to inhale through one nostril and then exhale through the other.

Technique #3 – Focused-Intention Breath Work

For this technique, think of what you want more of and what you want to rid yourself of.

Then name each inhale and each exhale. Let the words flow easily and don't worry about which words you select. They may change with each breath or remain the same. By allowing the words to flow, you may be surprised at some of the things you are trying to let go of!

As you inhale, say silently, "I am breathing in calm (peace, serenity," etc.)

As you exhale, say silently, "I am breathing out tension (stress, worry," etc.)

Technique #4 – The Aaahhh Breath

This is my favorite technique. I learned it at a wonderful retreat center, PeaceWeavers*. I have used it at the office occasionally, only to have my co-workers stare at me and wonder what in the world I'm doing.

By using the sound of "aaahhh," we relax our jaws and the muscles in our faces. When we are stressed, we tend to clench our jaws and squint our eyes, so we need to consciously relax these muscles to release the tension. By using a sound, we also empty our lungs completely, which allows us to inhale completely with our next breath.

Inhale deeply

As you exhale, say "aaahhh" until you can no longer make the sound.

Inhale deeply again and repeat until you feel calmer.

*www.PeaceWeavers.com

Now you have the first four tools in your stress-reduction toolbox. **Stress relief is only a breath away.**

Chapter 7

Tool 2: The Power of Thoughts and Visualization

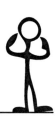

---

66 **W**hat the mind can conceive and believe it can achieve. **99**

Napoleon Hill

Our minds are quite powerful; thoughts and images flow through pretty much unrestricted 24/7, even when we're sleeping. Seldom do we "check in" or monitor what we are thinking or picturing, because the mind can run on autopilot.

Did you know that over eighty percent of our thoughts about ourselves are negative? We don't need anyone else to put us down as we do such a good job of it ourselves. Begin to monitor your thoughts and you will be shocked how many times one races by and reminds you that you are ugly, fat or unable to look good in hats.   Hey, we can't all carry off the suave, sophisticated Lady Di look. Some of us just end up with a bad hair day once we remove our bonnets.

Here are some other lies we tell ourselves:

"I should have made it to the gym today. I am just lazy."
"I am so dumb; I can't believe I made that mistake."
"Why can't I keep my mouth shut? I should not have said that."

When I listen to the words people use when talking about themselves, I am astounded at the constant put downs, questioning, judgments and criticisms. And these are the words that are expressed out loud. Imagine what the tape that is running internally is saying. Some of these words were programmed into our minds when we were just children. Someone we trusted said something about us, we believed it and the tape has played ever since. Thought monitoring is important, because it is from those thoughts that come the manifestations in your life. Napoleon Hill wrote, "If you do not conquer self, you will be conquered by self."

The other day, a gentleman asked me how he could stop worrying. His whole life he had wakened at night with worry and spent the day continuing to worry. It had become a habit he was ready to break. He knew that it did not make him feel better to worry, and it did not change the situation he was worried about.

Yet he fell back into this mental habit again and again. He challenged me to give him a tool he could use to stop the constant tide of anxiety that filled his thoughts.

"It is quite simple," I told him. "You have to have a contrary, positive thought to replace the destructive thought." Since you can't hold two thoughts at the same moment, when you find yourself with an old negative tape running, just put your hand out in front of you and say out loud, "Stop!" That will interrupt the thought (and startle people in the room with you.) Then replace it immediately with a different thought you have ready.

For instance, I used to worry about having enough time to get my projects done. I would wake in the middle of the night panicked that I had forgotten to tend to an important detail or that I needed to remember to make a phone call the next day. Any outstanding item was open to my scrutiny and worry. Consequently, I have learned to keep a notepad next to my bed. If I should wake, I simply write down the task, lay my head back on the pillow and silently say to myself, "All that must be done, will be done. There are no projects more important than rest at this moment. All is well." At other times, I say to myself, "Go back to sleep. You can't keep Johnny Depp waiting."

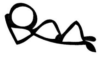

You can do this with any negative thought. Each time you exchange the negative thoughts, you create a more positive environment in your brain. Just by shifting your thoughts from negativity and worry to support and optimism, you can reduce stress. A lot of stress begins with a "worry" thought. If you can control those thoughts, the stress will disappear.

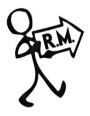

Mindfulness is one of the most important things you can practice. Being aware is being clear and being clear leads to becoming peaceful. So many people get stressed because they are uncertain what to do next or where their life is going. There are so many possible options, and they just want to know what to do. By quieting down the monkey-mind chatter, you can access the inner knowledge that is always present. Once you get clear, you can begin to block those annoying contrary thoughts that spring up out of fear, by returning back to your inner knowing and bringing your thoughts back into alignment with your peaceful place.

Let's Practice...

Close your eyes and picture the room you are sitting in. Not yet, don't close your eyes yet. If you do, then how will you know what the exercise requires? Envision where each piece of furniture is placed and where you are in reference to them. Imagine the colors, the fabrics, the textures of the room.

Now close your eyes now and try this. If the room is familiar, it was probably easy. Of course, there may have been small details you forgot to notice like a book or a throw pillow or the lucky troll doll you won at the carnival in fifth grade. Yet you were able to do this exercise without resistance.

By utilizing this technique, you can take a mini-vacation in your mind and create calm in your life, no matter the circumstances. Each of us has a place that brings up relaxed feelings. Perhaps it is a place where you spent a vacation—a beach or a cabin in the woods. Maybe you relax at the spa or in your comfy chair under a blanket. Perhaps it is a place you have never actually seen, but the pictures of it on TV or in a magazine mentally generate a calm, beautiful place to visit.

Once again, wait until after you read this paragraph, then close your eyes and picture that place; insert yourself there. Listen to any sounds that are around you. Are you alone or with other people? Are there any fragrances associated with this place? Are you sitting or standing? Mentally scan in as many of the details in this relaxing scene as possible. Pina Colada anyone? This will become your sacred spot for stress relief. This is the vacation spot you can return to without getting on a plane or behind the wheel of your car. Whenever you need to, you can return instantly just by closing your eyes and remembering.

Many people envision a place outdoors. They are at the beach or in the woods or in their garden, etc. Intrinsically, we know that nature heals. We feel good when we are outside. Perhaps it's because we are away from our desks, our computers and our phones. Of course, we could take our technology with us, but in this vision we have no Black-berry in our pocket. There are no texts that can break into our quiet, private, sacred moment. We can just "be." Think of it as a step back in time, back into the early days of history when there was no Facebook pokes, no texts, no instant messenger, no tweets, no IM - nothing to disturb your solitude. You know, step way back to the 1980's!

The next time you feel yourself getting stressed, stop the worry-thought train, close your eyes and go to your "vacation" spot. It only takes a moment to refresh, renew and revitalize. Banish worry, eradicate negative self-talk and get outside, even if only in your mind. Me? I'm going to the beach with Johnny Depp (on his private island.) Hey, it's my visualization and I can imagine anything I want to.

Exercise:

Write down in detail the place where you went for your "vacation."

Chapter 8

Tool 3: Get Moving

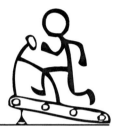

" Thoughts come clearly while one walks. "

Thomas Mann

I love to walk. It never fails to help re-center me and allows me the time and space to think and reframe issues I am facing. I know that I just do better if I walk each day. The small annoyances of life just don't bother me if I have taken a walk.

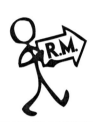

There is an old joke that says: What are the five words that strike fear in the hearts of men? Answer: "Honey we need to talk." It has been found that men respond better to conversations that take place when walking side by side than by face- to-face meetings. The intimacy of face-to-face makes some men uncomfortable, and they tend to close up and not share as freely. However, walking is less intimidating and the conversation flows much more easily.

I also love to walk outside in nature breathing the fresh air. There is something about being outside that energizes me in a way that a treadmill never can. I did spend one winter meeting a friend for mall walking. Normally I avoid malls as I dislike shopping. However the opportunity to exercise away from the winter snow and winds was inviting. That was the most expen-

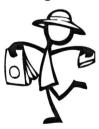

sive winter of my life! I would walk past a store and notice a sale going on. Hey, I would think to my-self, I really should

In our relationship, Bob and I walk and talk about life in general or any issues that are bothering us. We measure the severity of the problem in terms of mileage. "This is a two-mile issue," we say or, "This one may require six-miles." Luckily there are few challenges in our lives that required a marathon, but with every step we gain clarity and understanding by bouncing the situation off of one another.

stop there before I go home. I walked a lot that winter. I shopped a lot too!

When we are stressed we tend to stay immobilized. It seems like too much effort to get up and get out and move. Yet from a biological viewpoint, we are moving creatures. Our ancestors were hunter/gatherers. They were not TV watching/nappers. We were meant to move, and when we do, our stress decreases.

Physical exercise falls under the category of eustress. Temporarily, we place our bodies under stress by lifting that weight, running that mile or throwing that golf club after a bad shot! Exercise feels good. Emotionally, it makes us feel good about ourselves, and physically, we feel more relaxed and energized. Exercise also gives us time to set aside our worries, at least for a moment. When we focus on the moment instead of the money, the boss or the project, we are free to be in the "now."

Being in the "now" is the only place where we can be at peace. So much of our time is spent looking back in regret or looking ahead in worry. When we bring ourselves to the present moment, we are aware that right now, at this very moment, the reality is that we don't know what is going to happen in the future and we cannot undo the past. All we have is this moment and this moment and this moment…well, you get the idea, so get into the "now" now. When we return (to our home, our desks or our families), we are in a better mood to handle the tasks that are waiting.

Exercise doesn't need to be difficult. A simple walk around the block is a great start. Remember, this is about reducing stress, not entering into a marathon or a body building contest. Exercise can also be fun. Remember when we were kids? We didn't call it exercise; we were simply outside playing. Take a moment and think of the activities you loved to play as a kid. Climbing trees, jump rope, tag, four-square, hopscotch, touch football, hide and seek, ghost in the graveyard are all examples of the types of games we used to play.

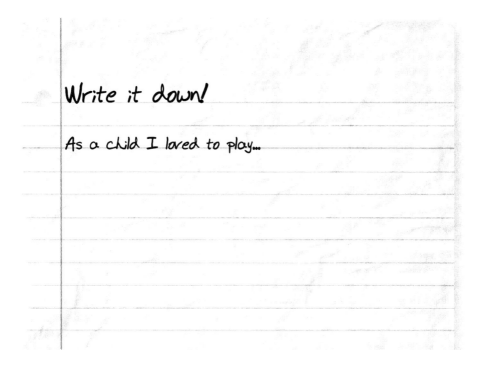

Write it down!

As a child I loved to play...

That child is still within you, waiting to play. Movement is not about competition; it is about feeling good. You didn't count calories or watch the clock when you were outside playing, except to know when you had to stop to go inside for dinner. Never once during a really good ghost-in-the-graveyard game with neighborhood friends did I stop and say, "Sorry I have now done my thirty minutes of exercise, and am going inside to get some work done."

When children play, they relieve whatever stress they have. That is why recess was so important to our school day. It was the time when we could relax, turn off our "thinking" brains and let our bodies move. We could talk with friends, let off steam and prepare ourselves for the next few hours of sitting in a classroom. If it makes such good sense for children, why do we stop it when we grow up!?

Think about what you can do each day to get your body moving. You already know what you should do, but what are you actually doing? In order to get the stress-relieving benefit of exercise, you need an Exercise Plan of Action—an EPOA. Make a list of things you can do every day when stress is present or to prevent stress from gaining an advantage. Remember to create this list engaging your "child-brain" memories of games you loved to play. Anyone want to join me in a game of Chinese jump rope?

EPOA Exercise:

I will remember to do at least one of the following activities every day:

Just in case you are not yet convinced that exercise can be fun, consider this:

A passionate kiss can burn six calories per minute!

Still not convinced that you can do whatever you make up your mind to do? Consider running (or walking) in a marathon (26.2 miles). While in my forties, I have completed two marathons. What an exhilarating feeling it was to cross that finish line and know that I had accomplished a personal goal that took months of training! Truth be told, my attitude at mile 23 was a little more along the lines of, "What was I thinking?"

But it is not the physical preparation that conquers. It is the mental chatter that makes the difference between stopping and going on. Many people on the course talk themselves out of the race. The messages we give ourselves are far more powerful than the messages that come from others. We believe ourselves!

"My feet hurt."
"I'm tired."
"I'm just going to sit down and rest for a minute or two at the next mile marker."
"It's hot."
"I'm hungry."
"This is too hard."

You get the idea. A blister didn't force the person to abandon the goal, the inner chatter that they allowed did it! Each excuse, compounded by belief, persuaded them to give up on their goals and achieve their dreams.

Conversely, I also watched people who talked themselves into continuing.
"I can make it to the next mile marker."
"My feet hurt, but I can deal with them back at the hotel."

"This pain is nothing compared to what cancer patients are going through. If they can make it through their treatments, I can make it through this race."

"I walk for my mother, my father…"

The difference between those who cross the finish line and those who don't is the state of their minds, not the condition of their bodies. We can convince ourselves about the truth of any story. We can talk ourselves into, or out of, almost anything. We can also convince our "inner knowing" that whatever we choose, we can complete—and that includes living a stress-free life.

Chapter 9

Tool 4: Journal

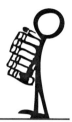

❝ Journal writing
is a voyage to the interior. **❞**

Christina Baldwin

Write it down. Get it out. Verbalize freely on paper. Use this tool when you want clarity and privacy. No one needs to see what you have written—you don't even have to save it if you don't want to—but there are enormous benefits in writing out whatever is bothering you.

There are many ways to journal, but no single method is the best. Choose the one that feels best to you. You can sit down at your computer keyboard and type until you run out of words, or you can pick up a pen or pencil and write in a notebook. You can journal every day or just when something is upsetting you. Journaling is really easy, and yet so many people avoid doing it. Try it and discover for yourself if it is right for you.

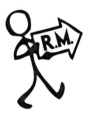

The infinite monkey theorem states that if a monkey hits keys at random on a keyboard for an infinite amount of time, they will eventually write something recognizable, like a work by Shakespeare or Paris Hilton. While scientists have yet to be able to test the theory through infinity there was a group of enterprising young students who procured a grant to test the theory. Apparently these particular monkeys suffered writer's block as they barely produced any letters and no recognizable words. They did, however, use the computer keyboard as a toilet frequently, leading me to believe that they may have been literary critics rather than authors!

Let's Get Started...

Often when we are facing an issue that is creating stress in our lives, we only look at it from our ego's point of view. "I am right and (he, she, it) is wrong." We may tell ourselves that if only the other person would change, or if the circumstances were different, we would feel better. Then, all would be right in our world. However, it is not easy to change the world to suit our needs, and when we are willing to broaden our perceptions, we can often find peace within the storm.

Once, when I was in a women's group, I began to ask questions during a meeting. I asked a woman there about the job she did for the organization. Actually, I only wanted to know what she did, how she did it and what the process was. Clearly, she felt attacked by my questions, and she became defensive and very rude to me. I left the meeting feeling verbally abused and very upset.

Back at home my thoughts (ego) kept telling me that if I could get this woman to leave the organization, it would make me happy. When I began to journal my feelings about the experience, the following phrase suddenly jumped out of my writing: "Even the timid, shy mouse will bite when it's cornered." That phrase challenged my thinking, so I began to examine it more closely.

It is true that this woman was usually quite quiet and sweet, so why did she feel cornered by my questions? Did she think that I wanted to take her job away from her and do it myself? Did she think I was implying that she did not do a good job? Had she felt cornered so she fought back defensively?

Putting down my pen, I picked up the phone and called her. I apologized if she felt attacked by my questions and assured her that I did not covet her job. I reassured her that my only goal was to understand more about what she did. Her voice softened and she began to tell me all about all the things she had achieved for the organization. It was evident in her voice how proud she was of her work. It ended up being a great conversation that turned into a very close friendship. What could have been a negative and destructive situation was resolved in a positive and wonderful way, because I had been able to get in touch with my inner feelings and to see it her way as well as mine.

When we get stressed about a situation, our minds continue to play a tape that puts us into a victim mode. Like that little mouse, we feel trapped, and we can get very angry. Though we may have no power to change the situation, we do have the power to change ourselves and our perceptions. Journaling can help this mental shift to happen, privately and powerfully.

Some people keep a daily journal. They write down the events of their day, including any observations or special moments they had. Those journals can create a veritable time-line and they are a valuable treasure to read again and again. Once, I was at a funeral where the deceased gentleman had kept a journal for years. His son read some of his dad's personal entries about his joy when he became a father and other special moments he had shared with his family. Hearing this man's own words and feelings being read at his funeral was incredible, and it was apparent how much his writing meant to the family he left behind.

Journaling for stress relief is more of a stream-of-consciousness kind of writing. Just write or type whatever comes into your mind, without regard for spelling, punctuation or grammar, until you have exhausted your feelings on the topic. Don't stop to read or make corrections as you go along, just let your inner feelings pour out. Later, if you want to, you can go back and "fix" what you wrote.

Finally, a school subject that I can use! Math was not my strong point, but English, being my native tongue, came easily to me. I may not be able to define a past participle or a predicate, but I can certainly use them in a sentence correctly. Journaling is not meant to be an English class assignment. It is not to be handed in for a grade or opened to peer review. It is merely expressing your inner thoughts and outer experiences on paper so as to gain a better understanding.

Whether you journal on a computer or with a pen and paper doesn't matter; one way is not better than the other. Just don't use disappearing ink, in case you want to go back and refer to your journal. If you do want to journal by hand and not leave a trace, then check out www.thinkgeek.com and check out their really cool KGB Disappearing Ink Pen.

Using pen and paper has a very different "feel." There is something visceral in taking pen in hand and feeling the subtle pressure of the pen against the paper. When you look back over what you have hand written, you may notice that your handwriting changed as you went along. If the words you used seem odd, but appropriate, this is another way to access your "inner knowing."

Also, using paper and pen means you can journal anywhere. You can sit in bed, under a tree, at the seashore (with or without Johnny Depp) - anywhere you happen to be. You can journal on a napkin, a notepad, a scrap of paper or in a fancy journaling book. The accoutrements don't matter; what counts is releasing feelings and gaining clarity and peace. You have the choice to either keep your journal or destroy it. But before you just wad it up and toss it in the trash, stop! Consider fire as a disposal method. An amazing feeling comes over you when you watch your troubles literally go up in smoke (just be sure to put safety first – remember, I have a fear of fire!)

I have used the "burn-and-release" ceremony at my workshops and witnessed the reactions of people as they let go of the things that are bothering them. I counsel them that they can either perceive the smoke as a release by burning away the situation, or they can picture the smoke taking their writings up to heaven so God can receive their troubles and help them.

A burning ceremony can be done at any time, but doing it during a full moon can be especially meaningful. Let go of what is holding you back or causing you distress and then write down what you would like in the month ahead before the new moon. Keep that paper until the next full moon, then burn it and let it go. As the cycle goes on, and the months go by, you can track your progress and see how your requests change. I have a friend who literally howls at the moon, but that is another story.

Another way to journal is to choose a phrase that is the direct opposite of what you are feeling. Instead of, "I am so stressed because I never have enough time to do the things I need and want to do," select a phrase such as, "I am so happy that time expands allowing me to accomplish both my needs and my wants every day." Write down your phrase over and over again. Some people write their affirmations fifty times each morning and fifty times each evening before bed. Others just write them down once and then repeat them aloud throughout the day. Writing and verbalizing "sets" the thought in your mind.

Post your affirmation in places where you will see it easily: the bathroom mirror, the computer monitor and the dashboard of your car are all good spots to hang up your affirmations. This way you will be reminded to state it aloud or silently throughout the day. I gave someone the affirmation, "Money flows to me from expected and unexpected sources." The next day, she went into a coat she had not worn in a while and found a $20 bill in the pocket! If you want to write an affirmation, just remember that they are positive statements, made in the present tense with gratitude. I am so happy and grateful that.....

Whether you use burn-and-release, or a computer and hit "delete," be assured that your words will never be seen by anyone again. (Especially if you are using a cool KGB pen) Nobody else has to discover your innermost thoughts unless you want them to. How's that for power?!

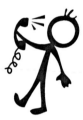

While journaling is a totally private activity, our next tool teaches you how to share your feelings with others.

Let's start writing!

Right now I am struggling with the following situation...

I feel...

What is my part in it?

Is there another way I can look at it?

Is there something I can do to change it?

Anything else?

Chapter 10

Tool 5: Talk It Out

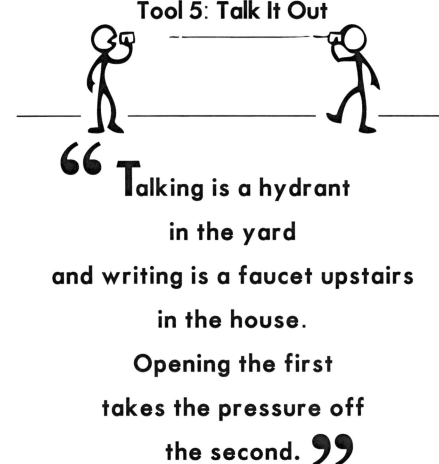

" **T**alking is a hydrant

in the yard

and writing is a faucet upstairs

in the house.

Opening the first

takes the pressure off

the second. "

Robert Frost

Mr. Frost seems to be implying that it is easier to talk than to write, and most of us would agree with him. Often, when we get upset, we immediately begin to tell everyone who will listen about the situation. Women, especially, use verbal communication to ease their minds. It just feels good to talk it out and be heard. But there is a caution before you begin to apply this method to stress relief.

There is a story about a man who goes with a great sage to the top of a hill overlooking their town. He brings along a feather pillow. The sage instructs the man to cut open the pillow and scatter the contents to the wind. As he follows this instruction, he watches the feathers float here and there as the wind catches and carries them. Some travel quite far, while others land in trees and bushes or settle into the dirt. The sage then tells the man to go and gather the feathers and put them back into the pillowcase. Perplexed, the man says that this is impossible, because the feathers have scattered over such a large distance. Some are inaccessible, and others can't even be found. "I can't do this task," he reports. Wisely, the sage agrees and explains that it is the same with words—once they are released, they can never be taken back.

Words are powerful! The old familiar phrase "sticks and stones" is not true. Words can hurt and hurt deeply. When we use words, we must always be aware of what we are saying and to whom we are saying it. Angry, annoyed or stressed words can erupt without being filtered. Just as an egg can't be unscrambled or a bell un-rung, words can't be recalled. Later, when we calm down, we may regret what we said, which a friend of mine refers to as "jumping into the pity pool!" We often succumb to the temptation to relate the tale as a "poor me" story and paint others as the perpetrators of our injury. So this tool, which can be extremely helpful, must be used with care and forethought.

If you have a situation that is bothering you and you call

a friend or corner a co-worker or sit at the dinner table with your family and begin to discuss it, stop! Begin with clear expectations by stating one of the following phrases:

"I just need to talk this out and be heard. I don't want any input or help. I need someone to listen to me so I am not talking to my Chia Pet®."

"I need your help on a situation I'm facing. Your advice and input would be greatly appreciated."

By being clear at the beginning, you will not feel frustrated when you just want to talk it out but are constantly interrupted by advice. On the other hand, if you want advice, and all you get is "listening," you may feel as if they are indifferent and don't care. If the "rules of the conversation" are clear in advance, you can usually get the support you need.

Remember to always choose your listening partner carefully. There are some people who will judge you or even turn your words against you. There are others who may spread the news (gossip) about what you share, or give you inappropriate advice. Selecting the right partner is the key to getting valuable guidance. It may be best to use this method with a trained therapist whose confidential insight can help you reframe and react in a more positive way. Whoever you choose, just be sure to start your conversation with clarity.

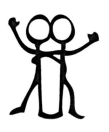

Melissa is my listening partner. I have been known to call her and start the conversation with, "Tell me that I am right." She quickly reassures me that I am, indeed, right and then goes on to ask if I want to tell her what I am right about. After I tell her the entire situation, she calmly asks me if I just want her to tell me that I am in the right or if I really want her opinion. Yikes! Talking it out can lead to all sorts of self-discovery, especially if you have a listening partner as bright as Melissa (or Frasier Crane).

Name names:

My listening partner is:

Because...

Chapter 11

Tool 6: Play

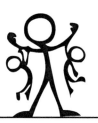

> ❝ **L**ook at me! Look at me!
>
> **Look at me, NOW!**
>
> **It is fun to have fun,**
>
> **but you have to know how!** ❞

Dr. Seuss

Now, I can imagine you saying, "Hey, this is serious. I don't have time to play." My point, exactly. Because stressful situations are so serious, is why you must start playing. Observe little children. They play all the time; they don't wait for recess or weekends or some scheduled moment that is labeled "free time" to play. Playing just comes naturally to them. They play, and they don't get stressed out. Inside of each of us is a little child who is waiting to play. If somebody would just give us permission, we could go there easily.

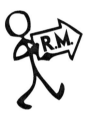

I can just picture you now, going up to your boss and asking if you can please go out and play. If your workplace truly embraces creativity, good health, high morale and low turnover, then you will quickly find yourself jumping rope in the lunchroom. Hey, Google headquarters has slides between the floors, pool tables, video games and more, and they seem to be doing pretty well on the financial front.

First, we have to understand what happens physiologically and mentally when we have fun. Both sides of our brains are engaged. We no longer live only in the left brain—the analytical, list-making, numbers, facts-and-figures side of our brains. The right-brain side is where our imaginations reside—the place of our spiritual connection and our intuition. (For more on this, I suggest reading Dr. Jill Bolte Taylor's book My

Stroke of Insight.) When we are faced with a problem, and we can access this region through play, we contact our "inner knowing." It has the ability to guide us and advise us in the action we should or shouldn't take. Playing doesn't sound so silly now, does it?

Playing also gets our immune system humming. We feel lighter and freer. We are in the moment, not somewhere out in worry-land. We breathe deeply and smile more. Our bodies relax, and our minds settle down. Children know this instinctively. How sad that we must re-learn this as adults. Peter Pan said, "If growing up means it would be beneath my dignity to climb a tree, I'll never grow up." When was the last time you climbed a tree?

In order to use this tool effectively, you need to be prepared before the stress strikes. When we find ourselves on the other end of an uncomfortable phone call, or get anxious about an impending situation that is not the time to stop and run to the "toy store." Toys must be accessible to us all the time. If we are ready to let go of the harmful-stress habit, we must have the means to make that happen easily available.

> **❝ I have a Pee Wee Herman bobble head on my desk, and when I need someone to affirm a decision, I just ask Pee Wee. He always agrees! ❞**

Try putting together a "Joy Basket." Fill it with small toys that can divert your attention from the uneasy feelings to the fun. Bubbles, clown noses, wind-up toys and stress balls are good starts for your collection. Have one at home, at the office, in your car and in your purse or pocket. I have a Pee Wee Herman bobble head on my desk, and when I need someone to affirm a decision, I just ask Pee Wee. He always agrees!

Toys can satisfy an important need: the desire to escape from feeling badly and returning to a place of joy and laughter. When I am stuck in traffic, running late or just plain lost I put on my clown nose and continue driving. Soon, my feelings of frustration evaporate, because, as I stated earlier, it feels stupid to be upset while wearing a clown nose! I also have one on my desk for when I am on the phone with a "cranky" person. They can continue to argue, yell and carry on, but I can maintain my composure and not take their tirade personally, because I have engaged my inner silly. Try having a fight with someone you love while wearing one of these—it can't be done. You have to stop yelling if you're wearing a clown nose, be-cause no one will take you seriously anyway.

When grownups play, we call it recre-ational activity. Some people golf, others bowl, some people play tennis or beat drums. They are all wonderful ways to reduce stress and have fun. However, to really utilize this tool, we must have a plan

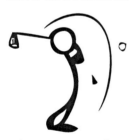

along with items that are quickly available at the moment of need. You can't just walk away from a stack of bills and hit a bucket of golf balls. You can't get up from an intense board meeting and immediately start square dancing in the hall. You need a strategy and some practical-to-use-gear that is available wherever you happen to be.

It doesn't matter which toys you use, or if you use toys at all, it only matters that you choose play instead of anger when you feel pressured and stressed. The other night, I took my daughter and her friend to a movie. It was rainy and cold, and we had to park in a space that seemed miles away from the entrance. So, as we made our long trek to the lobby, I skipped through the parking lot. My daughter looked at me with her familiar my-mom-is-so-weird look, but I did it anyway. It made the journey a bit faster, it was fun and I believe it was good role modeling for my child and her friend. We need to constantly be alert for ways to turn an uncomfortable situation into an opportunity to play. The circumstance may not change, but we will. And that will make all of the difference.

Exercise:

I will fill my joy basket with:

I will have toys ready in the following places:

Other ways I can play:

Chapter 12

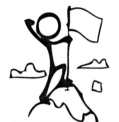

Tool 7: Take Action

> " **N**ever confuse motion with action. "

Benjamin Franklin

Have you ever had a situation so overwhelming that you felt frozen, paralyzed, immobilized? It feels as though you can't take a breath, because even that would require too much energy. Various options run through your mind over and over again, and you frantically search for the one that will take you out of this mess. Why do we turn to worry and mental anguish when action is clearly what's called for? Over and over we ruminate, while our stress levels soar.

When we choose to worry about a situation rather than do something about it, we place ourselves in the role of helpless victims, but victims are not happy. No matter what you are struggling with, you don't have to be a victim; there is always something you can do. Helplessness leads to hopelessness, and when people who are hopeless become depressed and full of despair, they lose all passion for life. This is not who you were meant to be.

You are:
> *Not a victim.*
> *Not helpless in any situation.*
> *Not immobilized.*
> *Not without hope.*

You are:
> *A powerful being, capable of creating positive outcomes.*
> *A capable being, powerful enough to change any situation.*
> *A clever survivor who can come up with a solution to any problem.*
> *A change agent, ready to take on each day with passion and commitment to who you are and who you choose to be.*
> *Faster than a speeding bullet, more powerful than a locomotive, able to leap tall buildings in a single bound.*

Well, maybe not, but you are super, man. (groan here)

Everyone can shift their awareness and change their life. I believe that everyone can choose options that are different from the ones they took the day before and find themselves heading in a new direction. The only way out of a situation is by determinedly going in, finding the best course of action and taking it.

Stressful situations often cause us to stumble emotionally so that we fail to think before we act. We are like an animal who is trapped and flailing about, trying to break free. But if we stop, take a deep breath and truly assess the situation, we can determine the steps to take that will be productive. We don't have to resort to hysterical or frenetic motion only.

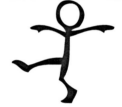

Sometimes, just taking one small step forward feels good, and it's a good beginning. When your desk is a mess and you're trying to get some work done, the stress just grows. The thought of sorting through all of those papers and establishing order from chaos is more than you can bear. You may work at the kitchen table rather than at your desk. You may find that you can just put your laptop on the coffee table and work from the couch. There are ways to ignore the issue, but ultimately every time you go to do some work, you are aware that the problem still exists. The stress is repeated over and over until you decide to do something about it. While you may not have the time or inclination to tackle the whole project right away, start with one corner or one pile or one drawer. The energy will develop as you progress. Over time, small actions will create big payoffs.

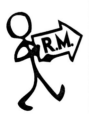

In Feng Shui clutter is seen as stagnant energy. So, if you are feeling overwhelmed and ready to make changes in your life, start with de-cluttering your home.

Just as stress can create inertia, taking action can build energy and confidence. Remember the law of physics: A body in motion tends to stay in motion, a body at rest tends to stay at rest (but not necessarily a quiet, stress-free rest!) This is yet another part of my education that I failed to completely grasp. Laws of physics to me are most useful when they are applied to how much pressure to exert when breaking open a bag of chocolate.

Sometimes searching the internet for information can break your log jam and move you forward. Make a phone call, meet with a key person, organize a project, make a list. "Starting" is the key to taking that first step towards resolution. As Nike® says in their ad, "Just do it."

Develop a Plan of Action (POA)

Think of a situation that is causing you stress right now and write it down:

Write down the results of these actions:

Write down the steps you have taken so far to handle the situation:

Are there other actions can you take to resolve the situation? (This is a good time to brainstorm and list any idea, even outrageous ones)

Which of these actions are most likely to bring you back to a place of peace?

What is your time frame for implementing these actions?

Develop your POA and write it here.
I am going to:

Chapter 13

Tool 8: Create

Your Environment

> **"** **I**'m a tidy sort of bloke.
>
> I don't like chaos.
>
> I keep records in the record rack,
>
> tea in the tea caddy,
>
> and pot in the pot box. **"**

George Harrison

While I don't advocate having a "pot box" in your home or office, I think George generally has the right idea. Clutter and chaos nurture stress. Have you ever tried to find your keys or an important receipt, only to turn the house upside down with no luck? Finally, after frustration, high blood pressure and popping-out veins, you locate the missing item in the oddest place you could never have imagined. Maybe the keys fell out of your pocket and ended up in your pajama drawer. Perhaps that missing paper was misfiled or stuck between two other papers. No matter the reason, when we can't find what we need when we need it, the result is stress!

Note to neat freaks:
You can skip down a couple of paragraphs—unless you want to feel superior to the messy folks out there. If so, go ahead and keep reading.

Organization is the first step to creating a stress-free environment. If you are so out of control that the last time you saw the top of your desk was when you first bought it, then stop and take a breath. There is a silly joke that goes: How do you eat an elephant? One bite at a time! When you have an elephant sized task ahead of you, break the task down into small, achievable steps: A drawer-a-day, just one closet, one room or your car. Shift one area at a time from disarray to dazzling. As you sort, file, clean and unclutter, you will immediately feel better and lighter.

As you do this though, establish a system that you can maintain. I once had a boss whose desk was constantly piled at least three inches deep with papers. Periodically, I was asked to help her organize her office. We sorted through each piece of paper and either made files to put them in, dealt with them right then or threw them away. As we got closer to the desk surface, we discovered receipts that had not been turned in for compensation, press releases that had not been sent in by the deadline and other important papers she had ignored, forgotten or searched for in vain. Hours passed as we plodded through the mess until, at last, her office was a masterpiece. Satisfied with a job well done, I returned to my own office, knowing that I had left her organized so this would not happen again, but no such luck! Within a week, the piles began to reappear, and in less than a month, the desk was deep in chaos again.

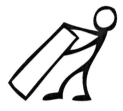

Her habit caused endless stress for her that reflected on her performance reviews. I could clean up, establish files and have a system in place, but I couldn't force her to change her poor habits for healthier ones. (I also couldn't force her to give me a raise, a paid day off or a business trip to the Bahamas.)

If you see yourself in this story, I urge you to create a system that you can live with. Living with clutter can be unrelenting, but it is better to deal with the mess regularly and frequently than to feel the weight of it as it accumulates. Don't allow disorganization's power to grow, while your own diminishes!

In fairness, I must note that there is one type of clutter that really doesn't qualify as clutter. There is a book about being organized where the author explains that there two kinds of people (no, not boys and girls.) Some live very comfortably with stacks of paper around them, yet they know where everything is in that stack. If they are looking for a receipt, they know exactly where to find it. They don't like file drawers, yet they can find anything they need. They have a high need to be able to "see their stuff." Those people are organized in their own no-stress way! Their system may not look like mine, but it works for them. They don't worry about finding something, because they know that is in the pile under the window, about two thirds of the way down. If they go into their closet and dig down about halfway through a particular pile, the black sweater will be right there. We can't rush to judgment about what "organization" should look like. If you can easily find what you need and you are relaxed, you're all right.

As my friend, Julie, recently posted on Facebook, "I just cleaned my house.... Well, actually, I just watched an episode of Hoarders, and now my house feels pretty clean."

Let's practice:

Evaluate your environment at home and work and make a list of what needs to be organized:

Now, place a number next to each area in the list above to determine in what order you want to tackle each project. Finally, make a commitment to your planning calendar a day and time to get the job done. But don't forget to put systems into place so the job never gets big and out-of-control again!

Neat freaks:
Start reading again here

Creating an environment for stress-free living involves more than just being neat. There are other elements that can enhance any space where you spend time. Aromatherapy, photos and flowers add up to a calm, inviting space. Think about 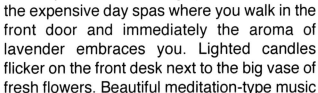 the expensive day spas where you walk in the front door and immediately the aroma of lavender embraces you. Lighted candles flicker on the front desk next to the big vase of fresh flowers. Beautiful meditation-type music is playing while you sit in a comfortable chair to wait for your appointment. Everything in the experience says, "Slow down and breathe." Just walking in the door has calmed you down.

Spas know that their environment sets the stage before the facial, massage or haircut even happens. One of these hectic days, I am going to walk into a spa and just spend time in their waiting room. When they ask if they can help me I'll reply, "No, I'm just having a stressful day and wanted a chance to relax. If you don't mind, I'm going to sit here for awhile, read some old magazines and soak up some atmosphere."

Studies have shown that just by looking at photos of people you love, you will feel calmer, so that's a good place to start, too. Find some pictures of family, friends and pets and display them in your home and office. Add a candle or two (a flameless variety might be better in an office setting). Use an aromatherapy diffuser, put pure oils on a cotton ball or burn incense. Choose lavender, nag champa, patchouli, vanilla - whatever you like - and let the air be filled with lovely, soothing scents.

Music can also be an easy shortcut to setting a mood. When you're cleaning the house, rock and roll! If you're working on a report, try some classical or meditation music. Do you need to get energized? Find something with a good beat. Feeling nostalgic? Oldies will do. Load up your iPod with music to fit your mood. At work, I tune in to on-line radio stations like AOL Radio or Pandora and select the genre I need to suit the work I have to get done. Music is a valuable tool to reduce stress. Something soothing will calm you. It works every time, so put your CDs in your car, load up your MP3 player, put a record on the stereo— you get the idea. Now when is the right time for me to break out my old 45 of Jive Talkin'?

Let's Practice:

Which elements do you want in your environment, and where do you want to put them? Look at the following list and note "yes," "no," "maybe" and "where."

	Yes	No	Maybe	Where?
Music	☐	☐	☐	
Flowers	☐	☐	☐	
Aromatherapy	☐	☐	☐	
Candles	☐	☐	☐	
Photos	☐	☐	☐	
Fish tank	☐	☐	☐	
Others	☐	☐	☐	

Chapter 14

Tool 9: Laugh

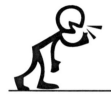
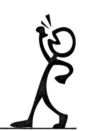

66 The time to laugh
is when you don't have time
to laugh. **99**

Argus Poster

My favorite stress relieving tactic is laughter. Laughter has been proven to reduce cortisol levels in the body. Cortisol a steroid hormone, or glucocorticoid, produced by the adrenal gland. It is released in response to stress…. Its primary functions are to increase blood sugar; suppress the immune system and aid in fat, protein and carbohydrate metabolism. It is the "fight or flight" hormone that helped our ancestors run away from dinosaurs. Dinosaurs are extinct now, but our need to be ready to get away from them is still present. What "dinosaurs" are in your life right now? Financial troubles? A difficult relationship? Health problems? Maybe you are just running late for an appointment or trying to put together a new toy that is "so simple even a child can do it." No matter the reason, our bodies react by releasing cortisol and helping us handle the "danger," even when the danger is only perceived, not actual.

Animals run, then rest. Humans run, then ruminate about what they were running from. We continue to ponder it, turn it over in our minds, victimize ourselves and tell our stories to any captive audience. Then, we wonder why we don't feel better at the end of the day. (When I don't feel better at day's end, it's usually because of the large pepperoni and anchovy pizza I had for lunch.)

A simple way to get into the present moment is to laugh. You can't be worried while you are laughing. You can't maintain anger, frustration, anxiety or any other low-level emotion when you are laughing. Try it right now. Put down this book and laugh. Did you do it? If so, you are on your way to bliss.

Laughter is a physiological action. You don't need a joke, a funny show or a person slipping on a banana peel to make you laugh. You have been laughing since you were an infant, and you can produce laughter at will. From a simple tee-hee to a full-blown belly laugh, releasing the sound will release the brain chemicals. The health benefits are enormous. Your immune system will get a boost, you will increase memory retention, your entire brain will wake up, your blood pressure will go down and your blood flow will improve. Breathe deeply, laugh and feel great!

Laughter is free, available whenever you need a break and it works! In situations where I am under tremendous stress, I drive around in my car laughing until I feel better. If you just burst out laughing at your desk for no apparent reason, people will probably give you strange looks, so if you can't bring yourself to laugh for no reason, turn to your Humor Plan of Action. Your HPOA is your "pantry" of things you can do to bring a smile to your face and a laugh to your belly.

I have asked thousands of people this simple question, "What is the one thing you do every day that is guaranteed to make you laugh?" (Sex doesn't count.) Generally, I get blank stares and questioning looks. They think and think but can't come up with a daily source for laughter. Eventually one brave soul will volunteer that she reads the comics in the newspaper or watches an old episode of I Love Lucy or Golden Girls. Hooray! At least that was one thing. But to be effective, your HPOA must have lots of ideas you can access wherever you are, because you might not have a TV conveniently available or a phone app with instant access to Chico and the Man.

Here are some ideas to get you started:
Watch funny television shows. DVR them, tape them, TiVo them or buy the whole season on DVD. Do whatever you need to have access to something funny anytime you need it. CNN is a great news source, but you will rarely walk away feeling giddy after watching it.

Watch funny movies. Go to the theater, search for them on the TVschedule, borrow them from the library, ask a friend to loan you one from his collection, start your own collection. Try NetFlix or Movies on Demand; there is never a good reason not to have something funny to watch.

Read the comics or any funny cartoons you can find. People fill my email inbox with funny stuff, and I save the best ones in a folder in my Outlook file. It gives me fun stuff to read whenever I feel stressed at my computer. My most treasured item was in-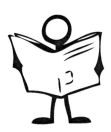herited from my grandmother when she died at 109 years old. It's a book she created by taping comics and funny news stories into it. Not only does it show me how much she valued humor, it also lets me see what kinds of things amused her. Consider starting a humor journal today for yourself (and perhaps for future generations.)

Watch animals. Pets can really make us laugh. They can slide off the desk, stretching and falling onto our keyboards (something my cat did a minute ago). They bring us into the moment and teach us how to relax. I remember during one of my moves, I was getting tense about all that I had to pack that day. When I saw my cat stretched out in the sun, napping, I realized he didn't have a care in the world; he was at peace and completely unconcerned about the move. Taking a lesson from him, I slowed down and relaxed. The work still got done, but I approached it with a renewed sense of calm. If you don't have any pets, check the internet. You will find many funny animal videos that people have posted.

Visit YouTube.com. It's my favorite stress-relief, laughter-inducing site. When I need a short, humor break, I go to www.youtube.com, type in the name of my favorite comedian and enjoy hilarious clips of their best material. I have also seen talking dogs and cats, hysterical bloopers and funny signs and photos. Humor is subjective, but I do not enjoy videos of people who get hurt falling down, crashing and other ways that are often shown on blooper reels. Pain does not equal funny in my world. Neither do photos that put down people because of the way they look. I am not amused by any stab at humor at another person's expense.

Hang out with young children. Pre-school kids can be really funny. They see the world differently; they haven't developed cynicism yet. They love to play and to involve grownups in their make believe games. It isn't easy to refuse when a little kid asks

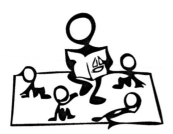 you to "play store" or build a Lego tower. Since laughter is contagious, just being near a laughing baby can make us laugh, as well. If you don't have a kid or two handy when you need one, go to YouTube and search for laughing baby videos.

Read a funny book or blog. When you find yourself threatened by stress, read something amusing. Keep a book of humorous essays handy or go online and read a comic's blog. Dave Barry, Erma Bombeck and others have written hilarious books that will make you giggle. If you don't have time for an entire book, just go online and read some of their quotes. Laughing out loud can be a quick fix for stress.

> **❝ My therapist told me the way to achieve true inner peace is to finish what I start. So far today, I have finished 2 bags of M&M's and a chocolate cake. I feel better already. ❞**
> *Dave Barry*

" **Bigamy is having one wife too many. Monogamy is the same.** "
Oscar Wilde

" Before you criticize someone, you should walk a mile in their shoes. That way, when you criticize them, you're a mile away and you have their shoes. "
Author Unknown

" One thing they never tell you about child raising is that for the rest of your life, at the drop of a hat, you are expected to know your child's name and how old he or she is. "
Erma Bombeck

" Whoever named it necking was a poor judge of anatomy. "
Groucho Marx

" **When somebody tells you nothing is impossible, ask him to dribble a football.** "
Author Unknown

" **Be careful about reading health books. You may die of a misprint.** "
Mark Twain

Develop your Humor Plan of Action:

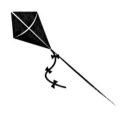

Chapter 15

Tool 10: Let it Go

> ❝ **S**ome of us think holding on makes us strong, but sometimes it is in letting go. ❞

Hermann Hesse

People think that letting something go shows a lack of power, but it is really the opposite. It takes a lot to let go and let God. It takes faith and strength of purpose to admit that something is out of your control. We are wired to be "do-ers" and "fixers," and sometimes we think that letting go is a sign of failure. It's not.

Since the results of letting something go can be instant, astounding and relieving, I questioned myself about why I find it so difficult to do. The answer that came to me was simple. When I release a situation, and I am prepared for any possible outcome, I have agreed to accept that whatever happens is for my highest and best. In other words, I am comfortable in having an end result that is not what I had hoped for.

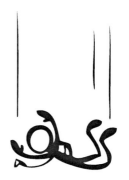

Think of it this way. You interviewed for a job you really wanted. You showed up with an excellent resume, well dressed and with articulate answers to every question. With that done, all you can do is wait and see if an offer is made. What you don't know is whether they also interviewed the owner's nephew or if someone from within the company also wants the position. It's a sit- uation over which you have no control. It's out of your hands, so let go of worrying about it. Be willing to accept that if you get the job, it was meant to be yours.

Also, be willing to accept that if you don't get the position, there will be another job waiting. Being hired for the first one, might have just impeded you from your higher destiny. Stay focused on what you really want: a satisfying job with a decent salary, surrounded by pleasant colleagues where you are convinced you can make a difference. If not here, then there.

Let worrying and self-criticism go. By accepting rejection as an indicator of new opportunities instead of failure, you stay connected to your highest ideals and your best outcome. Don't ever worry about not getting what you think you want, for in hindsight, you often see that where the road seemed to close, it was actually just an opening to a new journey.

Apply that philosophy to all situations. You are free to consider all possible outcomes, even those you may think you don't want. With faith, you can comfortably accept whatever comes your way. Faith is being comfortable in not knowing. If you already knew how things would turn out, there would be no need for faith. It is in the fog, that clarity often comes.

If you think you actually have control over your life, spend some time in a hospital emergency room. No one there thought they were going to have a day with such drama, but for one reason or another, they ended up in need of urgent medical care.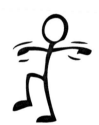

Unexpected circumstances happen all the time, so why are we surprised when they happen to us? Why me?, I think. But "Why not me?," is the more challenging question. Control is just an illusion. Release is a verb, an action we can take. When we release the reins of our lives, we find that things are smoother. When we stop trying to control people around us, we discover that they are capable of handling their own lives without our interference. We must stop trying to force situations into being the way we want and instead allow them to unfold in perfect timing and harmony. Life becomes quite simple when we let go of the need to have control and learn to accept that it is what it is.* Worrying about what it isn't won't change what it is. With this approach, stress dissolves and things are revealed in their own time.

* For more about this, read Byron Katie's book Loving What Is

The wind does not ask you to help it blow. You don't need to remind your heart to beat. The river flows whether or not you are there to appreciate it. Life happens with you or without you, so relax, let go and watch the miracles unfold.

Epilogue

People Look at me Funny

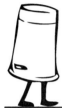

"Be who you are
and say what you feel,
because those who mind
don't matter and those who matter
don't mind. **"**

Dr. Suess

Whenever I give a talk, I often get the same comment, "People must look at you funny." They do, and I am the better for it. I live what I teach and my life is amazing. It's not that my life never has stress (in fact, right now I am typing this chapter on my laptop because my computer caught a very nasty virus that wiped it out.) If you are breathing, difficulties will show up sometimes. No one is exempt. The fact that drama happens is not what's important, it's what you do with it when it does that makes the difference between being happy and being devastated. Your choices are the key between being a survivor or being a victim, to be well or to be sick, to be a red head or a blonde.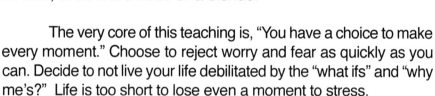

The very core of this teaching is, "You have a choice to make every moment." Choose to reject worry and fear as quickly as you can. Decide to not live your life debilitated by the "what ifs" and "why me's?" Life is too short to lose even a moment to stress.

People look at me funny whenever I:

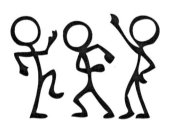

• Start dancing when I hear someone's cell phone ring with a catchy tune

• Wear a clown nose while stuck in traffic

• Play with my slinky at my desk when I'm put on hold for a long time

• Offer adults a chance to play with my wind-up, marching band or my laughing monkey

• Close off a nostril and take a deep breath

• Break out in spontaneous laughter at unexpected times and places

• Put on my cow hat and go out for a walk

When people look at me funny, I don't worry that someone will come and lock me up. Since I never drink alcohol, 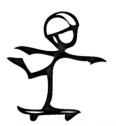 I am never drunk when these things happen. If some of the things I do are viewed as unusual or odd, I don't care. As long as my behavior is harmless, it doesn't matter what others think. I choose to be healthy and happy. I want life to be fun, and I want to find (and share) the joy in each moment. I live what I teach, because it makes me a better person. If people "look at me funny," it's because I'm doing something right, and I hope that, after reading this book, people will "look at you funny," too.

One last exercise:

What can you start to do right now that will cause people to look at you funny?

Write down your list here:

Chapter 16

Okay, This is Truly the Last Chapter

*In 3 words,
how do you handle stress?*

1.

2.

3.

I asked people this simple question. While I cannot advocate following their advice, they are fun to read. So here are their wonderful, wise and witty answers *(and my thoughts)*:

Drink more beer
(Surprised my son did not suggest this one)

Count my blessings

Serenity is mine...serenity is mine...

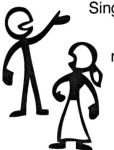

Sing show tunes

Praise-Preparation-Patience

Where's the chocolate?
(I like their thinking)

Eat more chocolate
(Ditto)

Laugh real loud!

Breath and Laugh

Faith, laughter & friends.

Make another choice

 Step by step

Read a book
*(Oh wait, you
already are!)*

Take a walk

Change the perception

Eat chocolate cake

PeaceWeavers, Breema,
Breathe

Eat, shop, breathe

Eat, Jack Daniels, cigarettes
(Not doctor recommended)

Sing to myself

Sing and drink

Clean, clean, clean
*(Come on over to my house
any time you want)*

Gnaw my elbow

I eat anything

I deep breathe

Drink, eat, exercise

Walk my dog

Go walk outside
(With or without your dog)

Take a holiday

Ease on down

Stop for prayer

Yoga class anyone?

Tai Chi immediately

 Cuddle your dog

Walk in woods

Cup of coffee
(I prefer tea)

Dance, Dance, Dance

Join laughter club

Weekly back massage
(Oh yeah)

Weekly foot massage

Just let go

Live, love, laugh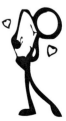

I love life

QiGong exercise
today

Bra/Shoes off
(This one works, trust me)

Friends, food, fun

Assess, regroup, overcome

Think calm thoughts

Pray for peace

Take a nap

Peace, be still
(Slow down, you move too fast)

Tears gently flowing

Laughter, tears, smiles

Breathe, think, sleep

Feel the breeze

Walk on beach

Dream, believe, transform
(Great plan)

Live, love, laugh

Peace be still

Focus on breath

Exercise and reading

Accept other's kindness
(Be a good receiver)

Breathe deeply. Repeat.

Eat, live, love

Look for laughter

Go have fun

Exercise while naked
(Yikes!)

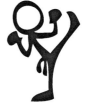

Look for laughter

Go have fun

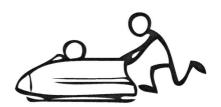

So, how would you answer this question? Go to my website, *www.TheLaughAcademy.com* and submit your 3 word tip. To reward you for your efforts, I will send you a bonus chapter with one more stress busting tool absolutely free. Now that is the deal of the century – you give me 3 measly words and I give you an entire chapter!

Acknowledgements

I must begin by giving thanks to Sharon. She is always ready with a word when I need one (usually something like aardvark or serendipity), also because whenever I ask her for a word, I always tell her that I will dedicate my first book to her. So here's to you Sharon, always ready to fill in the blank when I call.

I adore my children, especially because they are grown up and out of the house now, so we no longer get on each other's nerves. Kyle, Andrew and Lindsay (listed in birth order to prevent sibling rivalry) created enough stress in my life during their teenage years to develop most of the tools in this book. They are the light of my life and to say I love them would be too weak a word (I should call Sharon, she'd know the right word to use here.) It's not easy being my kid, because I am often doing something that embarrasses them in front of their friends, so I thank them for putting up with me and hope they are proud of their mom. I am certainly proud of them.

Parents. I have two – a mother and a father. My mother has supported me in every adventure I have pursued. She may not always understand what I am doing, but she is there for me every step of the way. Every book needs an editor and I have two of them. My father cannot read a sentence without adding commas in the correct places and reminding me that an auto accident that stops traffic is always ahead of you, so no need to tell the readers of this fact. "It cannot be behind you or it would not slow you down," he explained. So thanks for the grammar lessons and for helping me put the punctuations where they belong.

Of course, I also must thank my other editor, Andrea Gambill. She is a wizard of words and made this book what it is – readable. She took what I wrote and moved the words around and pieced it all back together again into its present form. It is said that a writer is only good as their editor and Andrea has made this speaker look like an author.

In this book I mention several stories that I attribute to my best friend, Melissa, so I must thank her for her wisdom, her humor and her ability to say stuff that I can use in my speeches. I always love when Melissa visits, because not only is she is a really good cook, I always get new material for my programs.

I have had so many mentors and teachers over the years who have helped me to become the person I am today (not that I am blaming you or anything). My heartfelt appreciation goes out to: (in no particular order, so don't get worked up if you are mentioned last) Steve Wilson of the World Laughter Tour, who first brought me into the world of laughter. Darcie Sims, my mentor in the field of grief, who encouraged me to bring my love of laughter into the bereavement industry. Donna Riegel, my "honorary mother" who was always there when I needed good advice.

There are many other people in my life who have encouraged, badgered and teased me (like my brothers David and Rick) into becoming a better me. To each of you who has touched my life and my heart, I thank you and ask that you forgive me for not mentioning you by name, but still hope that you will feel my gratitude and read the book anyway.

Finally, I must acknowledge my "honey," Bob. His patience with me, his tolerance of my crazy schedule and his love and support have allowed me to chase my dreams. We share the same sense of humor and can sing a pretty good, though mangled, version of Lydia the Tattooed Lady to anyone who will listen.

About the Author...

Nancy Weil began to laugh at a very young age. Soon after she discovered words and has not stopped talking since! With a degree in business and a career that has encompassed dog groomer, small business owner and Director of Grief Support for eleven cemeteries, Nancy has seen the difference that laughter can make in any situation. She is an officer in the New York State National Speakers Association and is a Certified Laughter Leader through the World Laughter Tour. Nancy has further certifications as a Grief Services Provider, Funeral Celebrant and Grief Management Specialist. She is an author, speaker, consultant and a pretty lousy cook! To learn more about Nancy and the programs she offers, visit her website: **www.TheLaughAcademy.com**

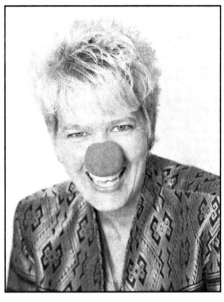

About the Graphic Designer...

Sandra Russo has a degree in Graphic Design and has worked on projects from logo design to magazine layout. She is currently living on bunk beds with her husband and dog in the back room of her mother's small house as they move from Western New York. They are in the middle of trying to sell their current house, move, purchase a new home, adapt to a new city and job, continue classes towards an MBA, and handle a family illness. Oh, and prepare for their first baby! In the meantime, she is using all of the tools that she learned in this book in order to not freak out.

About the Back Cover...

The people on the back cover truly understand the power of humor. The woman with the straw in her mouth is a heart transplant recipient. The group in the center are my co-workers and me at the cemetery. We are about to box and ship those clown noses to a charity called The Red Nose Institute (www.TheRedNoseInstitute.com.) They ship clown noses to our troops serving overseas. The gentleman in the hospital bed is about to have cancer surgery (he has made a full recovery.) As you can tell by their stories, life is not always easy, but that doesn't mean it can't be fun.

Scan this QR code with your smartphone
to visit the Laugh Academy online.

CPSIA information can be obtained at www.ICGtesting.com
Printed in the USA
LVOW061151100911

245706LV00003B/4/P

9 780983 656586